Handbook of Nursing Diagnosis

Lynda Juall Carpenito, R.N., M.S.N.

Nursing Consultant
Mickleton, New Jersey

Former Task Force Member
National Group for the Classification
of Nursing Diagnosis

J.B. Lippincott Company Philadelphia

London Mexico City New York St. Louis São Paulo Sydney

Sponsoring Editor: Diana Intenzo
Manuscript Editor: Kristen B. Frasch
Indexer: Eleanor Kuljian
Art Director: Tracy Baldwin
Design Coordinator: Charles Field
Production Supervisor: J. Corey Gray
Production Assistant: Barney Fernandes
Compositor: Tapsco, Inc.
Printer/Binder: R. R. Donnelley & Sons

Printed in the United States of America. For information write J. B. Lippincott Company, East Washington Square, Philadelphia, Pennsylvania 19105.

6 5 4 3 2 1

Library of Congress Cataloging in Publication Data

Carpenito, Lynda Juall.
Handbook of nursing diagnosis.

Includes index.
1. Nursing—Handbooks, manuals, etc. 2. Diagnosis—Handbooks, manuals, etc. I. Title. [DNLM: 1. Nursing Process—handbooks. WY 39 C294h]
RT48.C365 1984 616.07'5 84-12233
ISBN 0-397-54493-6

The authors and publisher have exerted every effort to ensure that drug selection and dosage set forth in this text are in accord with current recommendations and practice at the time of publication. However, in view of ongoing research, changes in government regulations, and the constant flow of information relating to drug therapy and drug reactions, the reader is urged to check the package insert for each drug for any change in indications and dosage and for added warnings and precautions. This is particularly important when the recommended agent is a new or infrequently employed drug.

To Olen, my son

for your innocence and wisdom
for our quiet moments and sudden hugs
for your unsolicited distractions
. . . I am grateful

for you are my daily reminder of what is
really important . . .
love, health, and human trust

Introduction

In 1973, the North American Nursing Diagnosis Association (NANDA; formerly the National Group for the Classification of Nursing Diagnosis) published its first list of nursing diagnoses. Since that time, the interest in nursing diagnosis and its application in clinical settings have grown substantially. In the 1970s, the main issue in nursing centered around the value of establishing a classification system for nursing diagnoses. Now that there is general agreement about the need for a formal taxonomy, the present issue centers around the implementation of nursing diagnoses. The challenge that nurses face today is one of identifying specific nursing diagnoses for those people assigned to their care and of incorporating these diagnoses into a plan of care.

This handbook is intended to help in this effort in two ways:

- By providing a quick reference to each diagnostic category in terms of its definition, etiological and contributing factors, and defining characteristics
- By identifying possible nursing diagnoses that could be associated with the major medical diagnoses.

Section I consists of 42 nursing diagnostic categories accepted by NANDA, plus three additional categories—Alteration in Respiratory Function, Impaired Social Interaction, and Potential for Infection.

Each diagnostic category is described in terms of

- Definition
- Etiological and contributing factors, which are those psychosocial, pathophysiological, situational, and maturational factors that can cause or influence the problem or health state
- Defining characteristics, which are a cluster of signs and symptoms that are observed in the individual with the problem.

A specific nursing diagnostic statement consists of two parts and reflects the present health state of the individual and the factors that have influenced that status. These two elements—health status and influencing factors—are represented respectively by the nursing diagnostic category and by the etiological or contributing factors. The relationship between these two elements is indicated by the phrase "related to." In graphic terms this inter-relationship can be diagrammed as follows:

Health status →	Related to →	Factors that influence the status
↓	↓	↓
Nursing Diagnostic Category →	→	Etiologic/ contributing factors
↓	↓	↓
Alteration in Nutrition: Less than Body Requirements →	Related to →	Anorexia secondary to chemotherapy

The diagnostic statement may be defined further by the term *potential* or *possible.* The use of a nursing diagnosis without the words *possible* or *potential* means that the problem has been clinically validated by identifiable defining characteristics.

Potential: A potential nursing diagnosis describes an altered state that may occur if certain nursing interventions are not ordered and implemented. Defining characteristics are not present, but etiologic and contributing factors are present. These nursing interventions are preventive in nature.

Possible: The word *possible* is used in nursing diagnoses to describe problems that may be present but that require additional data to be confirmed or ruled out. *Possible* serves to alert nurses to the need for additional data. Usually, defining characteristics have not been identified, and the presence of factors that can contribute to the problem have not been confirmed.

The presence of actual or possible nursing diagnoses is determined by assessing the patient's health status. To guide the nurse who is gathering this information, a Data Base

Assessment Tool is included in the Appendix at the end of the book. This guide directs the nurse to collect data according to the individual's functional health patterns. Functional health patterns and the corresponding nursing diagnoses are listed in the table that follows this introduction. If significant data is collected in a particular functional pattern, the next step is to check the related diagnostic categories to see if any nursing diagnoses are substantiated by the data that are collected.

Section II of this Handbook consists of seven parts: (1) Medical Disorders, (2) Surgical Procedures, (3) Obstetric and Gynecologic Conditions, (4) Neonatal Conditions, (5) Pediatric Disorders, (6) Psychiatric Disorders, and (7) Diagnostic and Therapeutic Procedures. Each of these subjects is represented by a series of major medical diagnoses under which are listed a group of associated nursing diagnoses and clinical problems. The intent of this section is to help the nurse identify possible nursing diagnoses in each of these areas. It is important to note that each nursing diagnosis must be confirmed or ruled out on the basis of the data collected. The use of a nursing diagnosis without clinical validation based on defining characteristics is hazardous and unsound, and jeopardizes the effectiveness and validity of the nursing care plan. The listing of tentative nursing diagnoses under medical and surgical diagnoses was intended to facilitate the assessment, identification, and validation process, *not to replace it.*

In addition to the potential nursing diagnoses listed under each medical category, there is a list of potential clinical problems or complications that may occur. Nurses intervene in both types of situations. The first type—medical or clinical problem—represents those situations in which nurses collaborate with other members of the health team in delivering treatment and care. Nurses do not prescribe the primary treatment in these instances, but are actively involved in the treatment regimen. These situations are clinical problems and are identified throughout Section II by the term *potential complications.* The second type of situation is the nursing diagnosis and represents those areas for which the nurse can legally prescribe the primary interventions. These items are listed according to the formal terminology associated with nursing diagnoses.

How to Use the Manual

1. Collect data, both subjective and objective, from client, family, other health care professionals and records. (Refer to Appendix: Data Base Assessment Guide.)
2. Identify a possible pattern or problem.
3. Refer to the Nursing Diagnosis List grouped under Functional Health Patterns (see the table following this introduction) and select the possibilities.
4. Refer to the medical diagnostic category and review the possible associated nursing diagnoses and clinical problems. Select the possibilities.
5. Refer to Section I and examine the defining characteristics of each possible diagnosis.
6. Are they present? If they are, complete the diagnostic statement with the specific etiological/contributing factors for the individual or family. If they are not present, go on to 7.
7. Gather additional data to confirm or rule out the diagnosis.*
8. If additional data collection is needed but must be postponed, the diagnosis is labeled as possible (*e.g.*, Possible Fear related to lack of confirmed diagnosis.)
9. If defining characteristics are not present but etiological/contributing factors are present, then the individual is at risk for developing the problem. Therefore, the problem is labeled as "potential" (*e.g.*, Potential Impairment of Skin Integrity related to immobility, dehydration, and incontinence.)

* Specific focus assessment criteria questions for each nursing diagnosis category can be found in Carpenito LJ: Nursing Diagnosis: Application to Clinical Practice (Philadelphia, JB Lippincott, 1983).

Nursing Diagnosis List Grouped Under Functional Health Patterns*

Functional Pattern	*Diagnosis*
1. Health perception–health management	Health maintenance, alterations in
	Noncompliance
	Potential for injury
2. Nutritional–metabolic	Fluid volume deficit
	Fluid volume excess
	Infection, potential for
	Nutrition alterations in, less than body requirements
	Nutrition alterations in, more than body requirements
	Oral mucous membrane, alterations in
	Skin integrity, impairment of
3. Elimination	Bowel elimination, alterations in: constipation
	Bowel elimination, alterations in: diarrhea
	Bowel elimination, alterations in: incontinence
	Urinary elimination, alteration in patterns of
4. Activity–exercise	Activity intolerance
	Airway clearance, ineffective
	Breathing patterns, ineffective
	Cardiac output, alterations in: decreased
	Diversional activity deficit
	Gas exchange, impaired
	Home maintenance management, impaired
	Mobility, impaired physical
	Respiratory function, alterations in
	Self-care deficit
	Total
	Feeding
	Bathing/hygiene
	Dressing/grooming
	Toileting

Nursing Diagnosis List (*Continued*)

Functional Pattern	*Diagnosis*
	Tissue perfusion, alteration in
	Cerebral
	Cardiopulmonary
	Renal
	Gastrointestinal
	Peripheral
5. Sleep–rest	Sleep pattern disturbance
6. Cognitive–perceptual	Comfort, alterations in: pain
	Knowledge deficit (specify)
	Sensory-perceptual alterations
	Visual
	Auditory
	Kinesthetic
	Gustatory
	Tactile
	Olfactory
	Thought processes, alterations in
7. Self–perception	Anxiety
	Fear
	Powerlessness
	Self-concept, disturbance in
8. Role–relationship	Communication, impaired verbal
	Family processes, alterations in
	Grieving (specify)
	Parenting, alterations in
	Social interactions, impaired
	Social isolation
	Violence, potential for
9. Sexuality–reproductive	Sexual dysfunction
	Rape trauma syndrome
10. Coping–stress tolerance	Coping, ineffective individual
	Coping, ineffective family
11. Value–belief	Spiritual distress

* The functional health patterns were identified by M. Gordon in Nursing Diagnosis: Process and Application (New York, McGraw-Hill, 1982) with some minor changes by the author. This nursing diagnosis list reflects the author's adoption of the National Accepted List. The author has deleted the listing of *actual* and *potential* next to a diagnostic category, because most diagnoses can be utilized as an actual or potential label.

Acknowledgments

I would like to thank the following people for their consultation during the development of the manual:

Rosalind Alfaro, R.N., B.S.N.
Graduate Student
Villanova University
Villanova, Pennsylvania
Staff Nurse, Intensive Care Units
Paoli Memorial Hospital
Paoli, Pennsylvania

Cynthia Balin, R.N., M.S.N.
Patient Care Coordinator
Orlando Regional Medical Center
Orlando, Florida

Ann Curtis, R.N., B.S.N.
Staff Development Department
Wilmington Medical Center
Wilmington, Delaware

Jacqueline W. Levett, R.N., M.S.B.
Pediatric Clinical Specialist
Wilmington Medical Center
Wilmington, Delaware

Mary Mishler Vogel, R.N., M.S.N.
Instructor
Helene Fuld School of Nursing
Camden, New Jersey

Anne E. Williard, R.N., M.S.N.
Director of Nursing
Delaware State Hospital
New Castle, Delaware

A sincere "thank you" to my diligent typists, Jennifer Jenkins and Maria Manel; and once again, to my husband Richard for his support on yet another project.

Contents

Section I
Nursing Diagnostic Categories 1

Activity Intolerance 3
Anxiety 5
Bowel Elimination, Alterations in: Constipation 7
Bowel Elimination, Alterations in: Diarrhea 8
Cardiac Output, Alterations in: Decreased 10
Comfort, Alterations in: Pain 12
Communication, Impaired Verbal 13
Coping, Ineffective Individual 15
Coping, Ineffective Family 17
Diversional Activity Deficit 19
Family Processes, Alterations in 20
Fear 21
Fluid Volume Deficit 23
Fluid Volume Excess 25
Grieving 26
Health Maintenance, Alterations in 28
Home Maintenance Management, Impaired 37
Infection, Potential for 38
Injury, Potential for 40
Knowledge Deficit 42
Mobility, Impaired Physical 43
Noncompliance 44
Nutrition, Alterations in: Less Than Body Requirements 46
Nutrition, Alterations in: More Than Body Requirements 47
Oral Mucous Membrane, Alterations in 48
Parenting, Alterations in 49
Powerlessness 51
Rape Trauma Syndrome 53
Respiratory Function, Alterations in 54
- Ineffective Airway Clearance 56
- Ineffective Breathing Patterns 57
- Impaired Gas Exchange 57

Self-Care Deficit 58

Self-Concept, Disturbance in 60
Sensory-Perceptual Alterations 62
Sexual Dysfunction 64
Skin Integrity, Impairment of 66
Sleep Pattern Disturbance 67
Social Interactions, Impaired 69
Social Isolation 70
Spiritual Distress 72
Thought Processes, Alterations in 73
Tissue Perfusion, Alteration in 75
Urinary Elimination, Alteration in Patterns of 77
Violence, Potential for 79

Section II
Medical Diagnostic Categories with Possible Associated Nursing Diagnoses 81

Medical Diagnoses 83
- Cardiovascular/Hematologic/Peripheral Vascular Disorders 83
- Respiratory Disorders 91
- Metabolic/Endocrine Disorders 93
- Gastrointestinal Disorders 101
- Renal/Urinary Tract Disorders 104
- Neurologic Disorders 107
- Sensory Disorders 116
- Integumentary Disorders 118
- Musculoskeletal/Connective Tissue Disorders 122
- Infectious/Immunodeficient Disorders 127
- Neoplastic Disorders 129

Surgical Procedures 132
Obstetric/Gynecologic Conditions 155
Neonatal Conditions 165
Pediatric/Adolescent Disorders 172
Psychiatric Disorders 194
Diagnostic and Therapeutic Procedures 202
Mechanical Ventilation 210

Appendix: Data-Base Assessment Guide 215

Index 221

Section I

Nursing Diagnostic Categories

Activity Intolerance

DEFINITION

Activity Intolerance: A state in which the individual experiences an inability, physiologically or psychologically, to endure or tolerate an increase in activity.

ETIOLOGICAL AND CONTRIBUTING FACTORS

Any factor that causes fatigue or compromises oxygen transport can cause activity intolerance. Some common factors are listed below.

Pathophysiological

Alterations in the oxygen transport system
- Cardiac
  - Congestive heart failure
  - Arrhythmias
  - Angina
  - Myocardial infarction
- Respiratory
  - Chronic obstructive pulmonary disease
- Circulatory
  - Anemia
  - Peripheral arterial disease

Diabetes mellitus

Chronic diseases
- Renal
- Hepatic
- Musculoskeletal
- Neurological

Malnourishment

Hypovolemia

Electrolyte imbalance

Situational

Depression

Lack of motivation

- Sedentary life-style
- Prolonged bed rest
- Stressors (*e.g.*)
  - Impaired language function
  - Impaired sensory function
  - Impaired motor function
  - Pain
- Fatigue, caused by (*e.g.*)
  - Sensory overload
  - Sensory deprivation
  - Interrupted sleep
  - Equipment that requires strength (walkers, crutches, braces)
  - Treatments
  - Treatment schedule
  - Medications
  - Diagnostic studies
  - Gait disorders

DEFINING CHARACTERISTICS

- Altered response to activity
  - Respiratory
    - Dyspnea
    - Shortness of breath
    - Excessive increase in rate
    - Decrease in rate
  - Pulse
    - Weak pulse
    - Decrease in rate
    - Excessive increase in rate
    - Failure to return to resting rate after 3 minutes
    - Rhythm change
  - Blood pressure
    - Failure to increase with activity
    - Increase in diastolic 15 mm Hg
    - Decrease
  - Weakness
  - Pallor or cyanosis
  - Confusion
  - Vertigo
- Impaired ability, related to fatigue, to
  - Turn in bed
  - Assume sitting position
  - Maintain alignment
  - Ambulate
  - Perform self-care activities

Anxiety

DEFINITION

Anxiety: A state in which the individual experiences feelings of uneasiness (apprehension) and activation of the autonomic nervous system in response to a vague, nonspecific threat.*

ETIOLOGICAL AND CONTRIBUTING FACTORS

Pathophysiological

Any factor that interferes with the basic human needs for food, air, and comfort

Situational

- Actual or perceived threat to self-concept
  - Loss of status and prestige
  - Lack of recognition from others
  - Failure (or success)
  - Loss of valued possessions
- Actual or perceived loss of significant others
  - Death
  - Divorce
  - Moving
  - Temporary or permanent separation
- Actual or perceived threat to biological integrity
  - Dying
  - Assault
  - Invasive procedures
  - Disease
- Actual or perceived change in environment
  - Hospitalization
  - Moving
  - Retirement
- Actual or perceived change in socioeconomic status
  - Unemployment
  - New job
  - Promotion
- Transmission of another person's anxiety to the individual

* Anxiety differs from fear in that the anxious person cannot identify the threat. With fear, the threat can be identified. However, fear and anxiety can be present simultaneously in an individual.

Maturational (threat to developmental task)

Infant/child: Separation, mutilation, peer relationships, achievement

Adolescent: Sexual development, peer relationships, independence

Adult: Parenting, career development, effects of aging

Elderly: Sensory losses, motor losses, financial problems, retirement

DEFINING CHARACTERISTICS

Physiological

- Increased heart rate
- Elevated blood pressure
- Increased respiratory rate
- Diaphoresis
- Dilated pupils
- Voice tremors/pitch changes
- Tremors
- Palpitations
- Nausea and/or vomiting
- Insomnia
- Fatigue and weakness
- Flushing
- Dry mouth
- Body aches and pains
- Urinary frequency
- Restlessness
- Faintness
- Paresthesias

Emotional

Person states that he has feelings of

- Apprehension
- Helplessness
- Nervousness
- Fear
- Lack of self-confidence
- Losing control
- Tension or being "keyed up"

Person exhibits

- Irritability
- Angry outbursts
- Crying
- Tendency to blame others
- Criticism of self and others
- Withdrawal
- Lack of initiative
- Self-deprecation

Cognitive

- Inability to concentrate
- Lack of awareness of surroundings
- Forgetfulness
- Rumination
- Orientation to past rather than to present or future
- Blocking of thoughts (inability to remember)

Bowel Elimination, Alterations in: Constipation

DEFINITION

Constipation: The state in which the individual experiences, or is at high risk for experiencing, stasis of the large intestine resulting in infrequent elimination and hard, dry feces.

ETIOLOGICAL AND CONTRIBUTING FACTORS

Pathophysiological

Malnutrition

Sensory/motor disorders
- Spinal cord lesions
- Spinal cord injury
- Cerebrovascular accident (stroke)
- Neurological diseases

Drug side-effects
- Antacids
- Iron
- Barium
- Aluminum
- Calcium
- Anticholinergics
- Anesthetics
- Narcotics (codeine, morphine)

Metabolic and endocrine disorders
- Anorexia nervosa
- Obesity
- Hypothyroidism
- Hyperparathyroidism

Pain (upon defecation)
- Hemorrhoids
- Back injury

Decreased peristalsis related to hypoxia (cardiac, pulmonary)

Situational

Immobility
Pregnancy
Stress
Lack of privacy
Inadequate diet (lack of roughage/thiamine)

Surgery
Lack of exercise
Irregular evacuation patterns
Dehydration
Habitual laxative use
Fear of rectal or cardiac pain

Maturational

Infant: Formula
Child: Toilet training (reluctance to interrupt play)
Elderly: Decreased motility of GI tract

DEFINING CHARACTERISTICS

Hard, formed stool
Decreased bowel sounds
Defecation occurs less than three times a week
Reported feeling of rectal fullness
Reported feeling of pressure in rectum
Straining and pain on defecation
Palpable impaction

Bowel Elimination, Alterations In: Diarrhea

DEFINITION

Diarrhea: The state in which the individual experiences or is at high risk of experiencing frequent passage of liquid stool or unformed stool.

ETIOLOGICAL AND CONTRIBUTING FACTORS

Pathophysiological

Nutritional disorders and malabsorptive syndromes
- Kwashiorkor
- Gastritis
- Peptic ulcer
- Diverticulitis
- Ulcerative colitis
- Crohn's disease
- Lactose intolerance
- Spastic colon
- Celiac disease (sprue)
- Irritable bowel

- Metabolic and endocrine disorders
  - Diabetes mellitus
  - Thyrotoxicosis
  - Addison's disease
- Dumping syndrome
- Infectious process
  - Trichinosis
  - Dysentery
  - Cholera
  - Malaria
  - Shigellosis
  - Typhoid fever
  - Infectious hepatitis
- Cancer
- Uremia
- Tuberculosis
- Arsenic poisoning
- Fecal impaction
- Surgical intervention of the bowel (Loss of bowel, ileal bypass)

Situational

- Stress or anxiety
- Irritating foods (fruits, bran cereals)
- Tube feedings
- Travel
  - Change in bacteria in water
  - Bacteria, virus, parasite to which no immunity is present
- Hot weather
- Increased caffeine consumption
- Chemotherapy
- Drug side-effects
  - Thyroid agents
  - Antacids
  - Laxatives
  - Stool softeners
  - Antibiotics

Maturational

- Allergies
  - Infant: Breast-fed babies
  - Elderly: Decreased sphincter reflexes

DEFINING CHARACTERISTICS

- Loose, liquid stools
- Increased frequency (more than three a day)
- Urgency

Cramping/abdominal pain
Increased frequency of bowel sounds
Increase in fluidity or volume of stools

Cardiac Output, Alterations In: Decreased: (specify)

DEFINITION

Alterations in Cardiac Output: Decreased: A state in which the individual experiences a reduction in the amount of blood pumped by the heart, resulting in compromised cardiac function.

Note: The use of this diagnostic category will not cover the treatment of decreased cardiac output (which is a clinical problem) but will focus on the functional abilities of the individual that are compromised because of decreased cardiac output. To represent this relationship, the diagnosis will be linked with the compromised functional abilities by means of a colon (:) and not by the phrase *related to.* The phrase *related to,* as in *Alterations in Cardiac Output Related to Congestive Heart Failure,* would refer to a clinical situation that is more in the realm of medicine than the realm of nursing. Because the nurse can diagnose and treat *responses* to decreased cardiac output, the diagnosis can be structured as *Alterations in Cardiac Output: Decreased: Activity Intolerance Secondary to Myocardial Ischemia.*

ETIOLOGICAL AND CONTRIBUTING FACTORS

Pathophysiological

Cardiac factors
- Bradycardia
- Tachycardia
- Congestive heart failure
- Cardiogenic shock

- Heart block
- Reduced stroke volume
- Myocardial infarction
- Valvular stenosis or insufficiency
- Hypertension

Pulmonary disorders

- Chronic obstructive pulmonary disease
- COR pulmonale
- Congestive heart failure

Endocrine disorders

- Adrenocortical insufficiency
- Hypothyroidism
- Diabetes mellitus

Hematological disorders

- Polycythemia
- Anemia
- Clotting alterations

Fluid and electrolyte imbalances

- Hypo- or hypercalcemia
- Hypo- or hyperkalemia
- Hypo- or hypervolemia

Situational

- Shock
- Vagal stimulation
- Starvation
- Sepsis
- Hypo- or hyperthermia
- Stress
- Dialysis
- Surgery, anesthesia
- Medications
  - Diuretics
  - Antihypertensives
  - Vasoconstrictors
  - Vasodilators
- Allergic response

Maturational

Newborn/infant

- Tetrology of Fallot
- Septal defects
- Patent ductus arteriosus
- Valvular defects
- Coarctation of the aorta

DEFINING CHARACTERISTICS

- Low blood pressure
- Rapid pulse
- Restlessness
- Dysrhythmia
- Oliguria
- Fatigability

Cyanosis
Dyspnea
Angina
Vertigo
Edema (peripheral, sacral)

Comfort, Alterations in: Pain

DEFINITION

Alterations in Comfort: Pain: A state in which the individual experiences an uncomfortable sensation in response to a noxious stimulus.

ETIOLOGICAL AND CONTRIBUTING FACTORS

Any factor can contribute to alterations in comfort. The most common are listed below.

Pathophysiological

- Musculoskeletal disorders
  - Fractures
  - Contractures
  - Spasms
  - Arthritis
  - Spinal cord disorders
- Visceral disorders
  - Cardiac
  - Renal
  - Intestinal
  - Pulmonary
- Cancer
- Vascular disorders
  - Vasospasm
  - Occlusion
  - Phlebitis
  - Vasodilation (headache)
- Inflammation
  - Nerve
  - Tendon
  - Bursa
  - Joint
  - Muscle

Situational

- Trauma (surgery, accidents)
- Diagnostic tests
  - Venipuncture
  - Biopsy

Invasive scanning (*e.g.*, IVP)
Immobility/improper positioning
Overactivity
Pressure points (tight cast, Ace bandage)
Pregnancy (prenatal, intrapartem, postpartem)

DEFINING CHARACTERISTICS

The person reports pain (may be the only defining characteristic present)
Autonomic response in acute pain
Blood pressure increased
Pulse increased
Respirations increased
Diaphoresis
Dilated pupils
Guarded position
Facial mask of pain
Crying, moaning

Communication, Impaired Verbal

DEFINITION

Impaired Verbal Communication: The state in which the individual experiences, or could experience, a decreased ability to speak appropriately or understand the meaning of words.

ETIOLOGICAL AND CONTRIBUTING FACTORS

Pathophysiological

Cerebral impairment
Expressive or receptive aphasia
Cerebrovascular accident
Brain damage (*e.g.*, birth/head trauma)

- CNS depression/increased intracranial pressure
- Tumor (of the head, neck, or spinal cord)
- Mental retardation
- Chronic hypoxia/decreased cerebral blood flow

Neurologic impairment
- Quadriplegia
- Nervous system diseases (*e.g.*, myasthenia gravis, multiple sclerosis)
- Vocal cord paralysis

Respiratory impairment (*e.g.*, shortness of breath)
Auditory impairment (decreased hearing)
Laryngeal edema/infection

Situational

Surgery
- Endotracheal intubation
- Tracheostomy/tracheotomy/laryngectomy
- Surgery of the head, face, neck, or mouth

Pain (especially of the mouth or throat)
Drugs (*e.g.*, CNS depressants, anesthesia)
Oral deformities
- Cleft lip or palate
- Malocclusion or fractured jaw
- Missing teeth

Speech pathology
- Stuttering
- Lisping
- Ankyglosia ("tongue-tie")
- Voice problems

Language barrier (unfamiliar language or dialect)
Psychological barrier (*e.g.*, fear, shyness)
Lack of privacy
Lack of support system

DEFINING CHARACTERISTICS

Stuttering
Slurring
Problem in finding the correct word when speaking
Weak or absent voice
Shortness of breath, ineffective breathing pattern
Decreased auditory comprehension
Deafness or inattention to noises or voices

Articulation or motor planning problems (*i.e.*, difficulty forming words, making sentences)
Inappropriate speech
Confusion
Inability to speak dominant language

Coping, Ineffective Individual

DEFINITION

Ineffective Individual Coping: A state in which the individual experiences, or is at risk of experiencing, an inability to manage internal or environmental stressors adequately due to inadequate resources (physical, psychological, or behavioral).

ETIOLOGICAL AND CONTRIBUTING FACTORS

Pathophysiological

Changes in body integrity
- Loss of body part
- Disfigurement secondary to trauma or surgery
- Altered appearance due to drugs, radiation, or other treatment

Altered affect caused by changes in body chemistry
- Tumor (brain)
- Hormonal treatment
- Injection of mood-altering substance

Physiological manifestations of persistent stress

Situational

Changes in physical environment
- War
- Natural disaster
- Relocation
- Seasonal work (migrant worker)
- Poverty

Disruption of emotional bonds due to
- Death
- Relocation

- Separation or divorce
- Desertion
- Hospitalization
- Incarceration

Unsatisfactory support system

Institutionalization

- Jail
- Foster home
- Orphanage
- Nursing home
- Educational institution
- Maintenance institution for disabled

Sensory overload

- Critical care unit
- Factory environment
- Urbanization: crowding, noise pollution, excessive activity

Inadequate psychological resources

- Poor self esteem
- Excessive negative beliefs about self
- Helplessness
- Lack of motivation to respond

Culturally-related conflicts with life experiences

- Premarital sex
- Abortion
- Need for medical intervention (*e.g.*, Christian Scientist)

Maturational

Child

- Developmental tasks (independence vs dependence)
- Entry into school
- Competition among peers
- Peer relationships

Adolescent

- Physical and emotional changes
- Independence from family
- Heterosexual relationships
- Sexual awareness
- Educational demands
- Career choices

Young adult

- Career choices
- Educational demands
- Leaving home
- Marriage
- Parenthood

Middle adult

- Physical signs of aging
- Career pressures
- Child-rearing problems
- Problems with relatives
- Social status needs
- Aging parents

Elderly

- Physical changes
- Retirement

Changes in financial status
Change in residence
Response of others to older people

DEFINING CHARACTERISTICS

Verbalization of inability to cope
Distortion or confusion of roles
Inability to meet basic needs
Inability to make decisions
Inability to ask for help
Destructive behavior toward self or others
Change in usual communication patterns
Inappropriate use of defense mechanisms
Frequent illness
High rate of accidents

Coping, Ineffective Family

DEFINITION

Ineffective Family Coping: The state in which a family demonstrates destructive behavior in response to an inability to manage internal or external stressors due to inadequate resources (physical, psychological, cognitive, and/or behavioral).*

ETIOLOGICAL AND CONTRIBUTING FACTORS

The following describes those individuals or families who are at high risk for contributing to a family's destructive coping behavior.

* The nursing diagnosis *Ineffective Family Coping* describes a family that has a history of demonstrating destructive behavior. This diagnosis differs from *Alteration in Family Processes,* which describes a family that usually functions constructively but is challenged by a stressor that has altered or may alter its function.

Parent(s)
- Single
- Adolescent
- Abusive
- Emotionally disturbed
- Alcoholic
- Drug addict
- Terminally ill
- Acute disability/accident

Child
- Of unwanted pregnancy
- Of undesired sex
- With undesired characteristics
- Physically handicapped
- Mentally handicapped
- Hyperactive
- Terminally ill
- Adolescent rebellion

Situational

- Separation from nuclear family
- Lack of extended family
- Lack of knowledge
- Economic problems (inflation, unemployment)
- Change in family unit (*e.g.*, new child, relative moves in)
- Relationship problems
- Marital discord
- Divorce
- Separation
- Step-parents
- Live-in boy/girl friend
- Relocation

Other

- History of ineffective relationship with own parents
- History of abusive relationships with parents
- Unrealistic expectations of child by parent
- Unrealistic expectations of self by parent
- Unrealistic expectations of parent by child
- Unmet psychosocial needs of child by parent
- Unmet psychosocial needs of parent by child

DEFINING CHARACTERISTICS

- Neglectful care of the client in regard to basic human needs and/or illness-related treatments
- Neglect of other family members (abandonment, desertion)
- Distortion of reality regarding the client's health problem, including prolonged denial
- Unresolved emotions of anger, depression, hostility, and aggression
- Verbalization of abuse by spouse

Hyperactivity
Helpless, inactive dependency of client

Diversional Activity Deficit

DEFINITION

Diversional Activity Deficit: The state in which the individual experiences, or is at risk of experiencing, an environment that is devoid of stimulation or interest.

ETIOLOGICAL AND CONTRIBUTING FACTORS

Situational

Monotonous environment
Long-term hospitalization or confinement
Lack of motivation, with signs of depression
Loss of ability to perform usual or favorite activities
Frequent lengthy treatments
Excessively long hours of stressful work
No time for leisure activities
Career changes (*e.g.*, teacher to housewife, retirement)
Children leaving home ("empty nest")

DEFINING CHARACTERISTICS

Statements of Boredom

Constant expression of unpleasant thoughts or feelings
Yawning or inattentiveness
Flat facial expression
Body language (shifting of body away from speaker)
Restlessness/fidgeting
Immobile (on bedrest or confined)
Weight loss or gain
Hostility

Family Processes, Alterations In

DEFINITION

Alterations in Family Processes: The state in which a normally supportive family experiences a stressor that challenges its previously effective functioning ability.*

ETIOLOGICAL AND CONTRIBUTING FACTORS

Any factor can contribute to an alteration in family processes. Some common factors are listed below.

Pathophysiological

Illness of family member
- Discomforts related to the illness's symptoms
- Change in the family member's ability to function
- Time-consuming treatments
- Disabling treatments
- Expensive treatments

Trauma
- Surgery
- Loss of body part or function

Situational

Loss of family member
- Death
- Going away to school
- Separation
- Divorce
- Incarceration
- Desertion
- Hospitalization

Gain of new family member
- Birth
- Adoption
- Marriage
- Elderly relative

* The nursing diagnosis *Alterations in Family Processes* describes a family that usually functions optimally but is challenged by a stressor that has altered or may alter the family's function. This diagnosis differs from *Ineffective Family Coping,* which describes a family that has a pattern of destructive behavior responses.

Poverty
Disaster
Relocation
Economic crisis
- Unemployment
- Financial loss

Change in family role
- Working mother
- Retirement

Birth of child with defect
Conflict
- Goal conflicts
- Moral conflict with reality
- Cultural conflict with reality
- Personality conflict in family

Breach of trust between members
History of psychiatric illness in family
Social deviance by family member (including crime)

DEFINING CHARACTERISTICS

Family system cannot or does not
- Meet physical needs of all its members
- Meet emotional needs of all its members
- Meet spiritual needs of all its members
- Express or accept a wide range of feelings from other family members
- Seek or accept help appropriately
- Adapt constructively to crisis
- Communicate openly and effectively between family members

Fear

DEFINITION

Fear: The state in which the individual experiences a painfully uneasy feeling that is related to an identifiable source (stimulus) that the person perceives as dangerous.

The responses to the perceived threat may be adaptive or maladaptive.*

ETIOLOGICAL AND CONTRIBUTING FACTORS

Fear can occur as a response to a variety of health problems, situations, or conflicts. Some common sources are indicated below.

Pathophysiological

Loss of body part
Loss of body function
Disabling illness
Long-term disability
Terminal disease

Situational

Hospitalization
Influences of others
Surgery and its outcome
Anesthesia
Treatments
Invasive procedures
Pain
New environment
New people
Lack of knowledge
Change or loss of significant other
Divorce
Success
Failure

Maturational

Children: Age-related fears (dark, strangers), influence of others
Adolescent: School adjustments, social and intellectual competitiveness, independence, authorities
Adult: Marriage, pregnancy, parenthood
Elderly: Retirement, relinquishing roles, functional losses

DEFINING CHARACTERISTICS

Feeling of physiological or emotional disruption related to an identifiable source
Feeling of loss of control (actual or perceived)

* Fear differs from anxiety in that the fearful person can identify the threat, whereas in anxiety, the threat cannot be accurately identified.

Associated Defining Characteristics

Increased pulse and respiratory rate
Increased blood pressure
Diaphoresis
Voice tremors/voice pitch changes
Increased questioning/verbalization

Fluid Volume Deficit

DEFINITION

Fluid Volume Deficit: The state in which the individual experiences, or is at risk of experiencing, vascular, cellular, or intracellular dehydration.*

ETIOLOGICAL AND CONTRIBUTING FACTORS

Pathophysiological

Excessive urinary output
- Uncontrolled diabetes
- Diabetes insipidus (inappropriate antidiuretic hormone)

Burns
Fever or increased metabolic rate
Overzealous dialysis (peritoneal dialysis, hemodialysis)
Shock
- Neurogenic
- Cardiogenic
- Septic
- Hypovolemic
- Anaphylactic

Fluid shift to extravascular space
- Ascites
- Pleural effusion

Infection
Abnormal drainage
- Wound

* This diagnostic category should not be used with individuals who are unable or not permitted to ingest liquids.

- Excessive menses
- Other

Serum electrolyte imbalance
Acid–base imbalance (acidosis–alkalosis)
Eclampsia (albumin loss)
Peritonitis
Diarrhea

Situational

- Vomiting or nasogastric suctioning
- Excessive use of
  - Laxatives or enemas
  - Diuretics or alcohol
- Imposed fluid restrictions
- Decreased motivation to drink liquids
  - Depression
  - Fatigue
- Blood loss
  - Overt (visible)
  - Occult (hidden)
- Dietary problems
  - Fad diets/fasting
  - Anorexia
  - High-solute tube feedings
- Difficulty swallowing or feeding self
  - Oral pain
  - Fatigue
- Climate exposure
  - Extreme heat/sun
  - Excessive dryness
- Hyperpnea
- Extreme exercise effort/diaphoresis

Maturational

- Infant/child: Decreased fluid reserve, decreased ability to concentrate urine
- Elderly: Decreased fluid reserve, decreased sensation of thirst

DEFINING CHARACTERISTICS

Decreased urine output or excessive urine output
Concentrated urine or urinary frequency

Decreased fluid intake
Output greater than intake
Weight loss (rapid)
Decreased venous filling
Hemoconcentration
Increased serum sodium
Increased pulse rate
Decreased pulse volume/pressure
Increased body temperature
Decreased skin turgor
Dry skin/mucous membranes
Thirst/nausea/anorexia
Weakness/lethargy/confusion

Fluid Volume Excess

DEFINITION

Fluid Volume Excess: The state in which the individual experiences, or is at risk of experiencing, peripheral edema.

ETIOLOGICAL AND CONTRIBUTING FACTORS

Pathophysiological

Renal failure, acute or chronic
Decreased cardiac output
- Myocardial infarction
- Congestive heart failure
- Left ventricular failure
- Valvular disease
- Tachycardia arrhythmia

Varicosities of the legs
Liver disease
- Cirrhosis
- Ascites
- Cancer

Time insult
- Injury to the cell wall
- Hypoxia of the cell

Inflammatory process
Hormonal disturbances
  Pituitary — Estrogen
  Adrenal
Steroid therapy
Effusion (abnormal fluid accumulation)
  Pleural — Pericardial

Situational

Excessive fluid intake (IV therapy)
Overtransfusion
  Blood/packed cells — Plasma expanders
Excessive sodium intake
Low protein intake
  Fad diets — Malnutrition
Dependent venous pooling/venostasis
  Immobility — Standing or sitting for long periods of time
Venous pressure point
  Tight cast or bandage
Pregnancy
Inadequate lymphatic drainage

DEFINING CHARACTERISTICS

Edema
Weight gain
Taut, shiny skin
Increased pulse volume or blood pressure
Increased venous filling
Intake greater than output

Grieving

DEFINITION

Grieving: A state in which an individual or family experiences an actual or a perceived loss (person, object, function, status, relationship) or the state in which an individual or family responds to the realization of a future loss (anticipatory grieving).

ETIOLOGICAL AND CONTRIBUTING FACTORS

Pathophysiological

Loss of function (actual or potential) related to a body-system alteration
- Neurologic
- Cardiovascular
- Sensory
- Musculoskeletal
- Digestive
- Respiratory
- Renal

Loss of function or body part related to
- Trauma
- Surgery (mastectomy, colostomy, hysterectomy)

Situational

Chronic pain
Terminal illness
Changes in life-style
- Childbirth
- Marriage
- Separation
- Divorce
- Child leaving home (*e.g.*, college or marriage)
- Loss of career

Type of relationship (with the person who is leaving or is gone)
Multiple losses or crises
Lack of social support system

Maturational

Loss associated with aging
- Friends
- Occupation
- Function
- Home

DEFINING CHARACTERISTICS

The person
- Reports an actual or perceived loss (person, object, function, status, relationship)
- Anticipates a loss

Associated Defining Characteristics

Denial
Guilt
Anger
Crying
Sorrow

Health Maintenance, Alterations in

DEFINITION

Alterations in Health Maintenance: States in which the individual experiences, or is at risk of experiencing, a disruption in his present state of wellness because of inadequate preventive measures or an unhealthy life-style.

Note: This diagnostic category should be used to describe an asymptomatic person; however, it can be used for a person with a chronic disease to help that person attain a higher level of wellness. For example, a woman with lupus erythematosus can have a diagnosis *Potential Alterations in Health Maintenance Related to Lack of a Regular Exercise Program.*

This diagnostic category can also be used for persons with acute conditions to describe other dimensions of their health. For example, a child with acute otitis media may have a diagnosis *Alterations in Health Maintenance Related to Lack of Immunizations for Age.*

ETIOLOGICAL AND CONTRIBUTING FACTORS

Pathophysiological

Not directly related to alterations in health maintenance

Situational

Loss of independence
Changing support systems

Change in finances
Lack of knowledge
Poor learning skills (illiteracy)
Crisis situation
Lack of accessibility to adequate health care services
Substance abuse (alcohol, tobacco)
Inadequate health practice
Lack of supervision for dependents (children, elderly)
Health beliefs (lack of perceived threat to health)
Religious beliefs
External locus of control
Cultural or folk beliefs
Alterations in self-image (poor self-esteem, distorted body image)

Maturational

See table below for age-related conditions.

DEFINING CHARACTERISTICS (in the absence of disease)

Skin and nails
- Malodorous
- Unclean
- Skin lesions (pustules, rashes, dry or scaly skin)
- Sunburn
- Unusual color, pallor
- Unexplained scars

Respiratory system
- Frequent infections
- Chronic cough
- Dyspnea with exertion

Oral cavity
- Frequent sores (on tongue, buccal mucosa)
- Loss of teeth at early age
- Lesions associated with lack of oral care or substance abuse (leukoplakia, fistulas)

Gastrointestinal system and nutrition
- Obesity
- Anorexia
- Cachexia
- Chronic anemia
- Chronic bowel irregularity
- Chronic dyspepsia

(Text continues on p. 37)

Primary and Secondary Prevention for Age-Related Conditions

Developmental Level	*Primary Prevention*	*Secondary Prevention*
Infancy (0–1 year)	Parent education	Complete physical exam every 2–3 months
	Infant safety	Screening at birth
	Nutrition	Congenital hip
	Breast feeding	PKV
	Sensory stimulation	Sickle cell
	Infant massage and touch	Cystic fibrosis
	Visual stimulation	Vision (startle reflex)
	Activity	Hearing (response to and localization of sounds)
	Colors	TB test at 12 months
	Auditory stimulation	Developmental assessments
	Verbal	Screen and intervene for high risk
	Music	Low birth weight
	Immunizations	Maternal substance abuse during pregnancy
	DPT, TOPV at 2, 4, and 6 months	Alcohol: fetal alcohol syndrome
	Oral hygiene	Cigarettes: SIDS
	Teething biscuits	Drugs: addicted neonate

	Fluoride	Maternal infections during pregnancy
	Avoid sugared food and drink	
Preschool (1–5 years)	Parent education	Complete physical exam between 2 and 3 years and preschool (U/A, CBC)
	Teething	TB test at 3 years
	Discipline	Developmental assessments (annual)
	Nutrition	Speech development
	Accident prevention	Hearing
	Normal growth and development	Vision
	Child education	Screen and intervene
	Dental self-care	Plumvism
	Dressing	Developmental lag
	Bathing with assistance	Neglect or abuse
	Feeding self-care	Strabismus
	Immunizations	Hearing deficit
	DPT, TOPV } at 18 months	Vision deficit
	MMR at 15 months	
	Dental/oral hygiene	
	Fluoride treatments	
	Fluoridated water	
	Dietary counsel	

Primary and Secondary Prevention for Age-Related Conditions (continued)

Developmental Level	*Primary Prevention*	*Secondary Prevention*
School age (6–11 years)	Health education of child "Basic 4" nutrition Accident prevention Outdoor safety Substance abuse counsel Anticipatory guidance for physical changes at puberty Immunizations Tetanus age 10 DPT } boosters between TOPV } 4 and 6 years Dental hygiene every 6–12 months Continue fluoridation Complete physical exam	Complete physical exam TB test every 3 years (at ages 6 and 9) Developmental assessments Language Vision: Snellen charts at school 6–8 years, use "E" chart Over 8 years, use alphabet chart Hearing: audiogram
Adolescence (12–19 years)	Health education Proper nutrition and healthful diets	Complete physical exam (prepuberty or age 13) Blood pressure

	Sex education with family planning, male/female Safe driving skills Adult challenges Seeking employment and career choices Dating and marriage Confrontation with substance abuse Safety in athletics Skin care Dental hygiene every 6–12 months Immunizations Tetanus without trauma TOPV booster at 12–14 years	Cholesterol TB test at 12 years VDRL, CBC, U/A Female: breast self-exam Male: testicular self-exam Female, if sexually active: Pap and pelvic exam twice, one year apart (cervical gonorrhea culture with pelvic); then every 3 years if both are negative Screening and interventions if high risk Depression Suicide Substance abuse Pregnancy (more than 18 years old) Family history of alcoholism or domestic violence
Young adult (20–39 years)	Health education Weight management with good nutrition as BMR changes Lifestyle counseling Stress management skills Safe driving Family planning	Complete physical exam at about 20 years, then every 5–6 years Cancer checkup every 3 years Female: BSE monthly Male: TSE monthly All females: baseline mammography between ages 35 and 40

Primary and Secondary Prevention for Age-Related Conditions (continued)

Developmental Level	*Primary Prevention*	*Secondary Prevention*
	Parenting skills Regular exercise Environmental health choices Dental hygiene every 6–12 months Immunization Tetanus at 20 years and every 10 years Female: rubella, if zero negative for antibodies	Parents-to-be: high-risk screening for Downs syndrome, Tay-Sachs Female pregnant: screen for VD, rubella titer, Rh factor Screening and interventions if high risk Female with previous breast cancer: annual mammography at 35 years and after Female with mother or sister who has had breast cancer, same as above Family history colorectal cancer or high risk: annual stool quiac, digital rectal, and sigmoidoscopy PPD if exposed to TB
Middle–aged adult (40–59 years)	Health education: continue with young adult Midlife changes, male and female counseling "Empty-nest syndrome" Anticipatory guidance for retirement	Complete physical exam every 5–6 years with complete laboratory evaluation (serum/urine tests, x-ray, EKG) Cancer checkup every year Female: BSE monthly

	Grandparenting Dental hygiene every 6–12 months Immunizations Tetanus every 10 years Pneumococcal annual if high risk, *i.e.*, Influenza major chronic disease (COPD, CAD)	Male: TSE monthly All females: annual mammography 50 years and over Schiotz' tonometry (glaucoma) every 3–5 years Female pregnant: perinatal screening by amniocentesis if desired Sigmoidoscopy at 50 and 51, then every 4 years if negative Stool guiac annually at 50 and thereafter Screening and intervention if high risk Endometrial cancer: have endometrial sampling at menopause Oral cancer: screen more often if substance abuser
Elderly adult (60–74 years)	Health education: continue with previous counseling Home safety Retirement Loss of spouse Special health needs: Nutritional changes Changes in hearing or vision	Complete physical exam every 2 years with laboratory assessments Annual cancer checkup Blood pressure annually Female: BSE monthly Male TSE monthly Female: annual mammogram Annual stool guiac

Primary and Secondary Prevention for Age-Related Conditions (continued)

Developmental Level	*Primary Prevention*	*Secondary Prevention*
	Alterations in bowel or bladder habits Dental/oral hygiene every 6–12 months Immunizations Tetanus every 10 years Pneumococcal, Influenza: annual if high risk	Sigmoidoscopy every 4 years Schiotz' tonometry every 3–5 years Podiatric evaluation with foot care PRN Screen for high risk Depression Suicide
Old-age adult (75 years and over)	Complete physical exam annually Laboratory assessments Cancer checkup Blood pressure Stool guiac Female: mammogram, sigmoidoscopy every 4 years Schiotz' tonometry every 3–5 years Podiatrist PRN	Health education: continue counsel Anticipatory guidance Dying and death Loss of spouse Increasing dependency upon others Dental/oral hygiene every 6–12 months Immunizations Tetanus every 10 years Pneumococcal, Influenza: annual

Musculoskeletal system
- Frequent muscle strain, backaches, neck pain
- Diminished flexibility and muscle strength

Genitourinary system
- Frequent venereal lesions and infections
- Frequent use of potentially unhealthful over-the-counter products (chemical douches, vaginal perfumed products)

Constitutional
- Chronic fatigue, malaise, apathy

Neurosensory
- Presence of facial tics (nonconvulsant)
- Headaches

Psychoemotional
- Emotional fragility
- Behavior disorders (compulsiveness, belligerence)
- Frequent feelings of being overwhelmed

Home Maintenance Management, Impaired

DEFINITION

Impaired Home Maintenance Management: The state in which an individual or family experiences, or is at risk of experiencing, a difficulty in maintaining self or family in a safe home environment.

ETIOLOGICAL AND CONTRIBUTING FACTORS

Pathophysiological

Chronic debilitating disease
- Diabetes mellitus
- Chronic obstructive pulmonary disease
- Congestive heart failure
- Cancer
- Arthritis
- Multiple sclerosis
- Muscular dystrophy

Situational

Injury to individual or family member (fractured limb, spinal cord injury)
- Surgery (amputation, ostomy)

Impaired mental status (memory lapses, depression, severe anxiety, panic)
Substance abuse (alcohol, drugs)
Unavailable support system
Loss of family member
Addition of family member (newborn, aged parent)
Lack of knowledge
Insufficient finances

Maturational

Infant: Newborn care, high risk for sudden infant death syndrome
Elderly: Family member with deficits (cognitive, motor, sensory)

DEFINING CHARACTERISTICS

Outward expressions of difficulty by individual or family
- In maintaining the home (cleaning, repairs, financial needs)
- In caring for self or family member at home

Poor hygienic practices
- Infections
- Infestations
- Accumulated wastes
- Unwashed cooking and eating equipment
- Offensive odors

Impaired caregiver
- Overtaxed
- Anxious
- Lack of knowledge
- Negative response to ill member

Unavailable support system

Infection, Potential for

DEFINITION

Potential for Infection: The state in which an individual is at risk for being invaded by a pathogenic agent (microorganism or virus).

ETIOLOGICAL AND CONTRIBUTING FACTORS

A variety of health problems and situations can create favorable conditions that would encourage the development of infections.

Some common factors are as follows:

Pathophysiological

- Chronic diseases
  - Cancer
  - Renal failure
  - Arthritis
  - Respiratory disorders
  - Hematologic disorders
  - Diabetes mellitus
  - Hepatic disorders
- Immunosuppressed system
- Immune incompetent system
- Altered or insufficient leukocytes
- Blood dyscrasias
- Impaired oxygen transport
- Altered integumentary system
- Periodontal disease

Situational

- Treatments/therapies
  - Surgery
  - Dialysis
  - Chemotherapy
  - Presence of invasive lines (*e.g.* IVs, Foley catheter)
  - Radiation therapy
  - Total parenteral nutrition
  - Tracheostomy
- Prolonged immobility
- Trauma (accidental)
- Postpartum period
- Contact with contagious agents (hospitalization, ill individual)
- Malnutrition
- Medications
  - Antibiotics
  - Steroids
  - Immunosuppressants
  - Tranquilizers
- Bites (animal, insect)
- Thermal injuries
- Warm, moist, dark environment (skin folds, casts)
- Inadequate personal hygiene

Maturational

- Newborns
  - Lack of normal flora
  - Open wounds (umbilical, circumcision)
- Elderly
  - Debilitated

DEFINING CHARACTERISTICS

- History of infections
- Altered production of leukocytes
- Altered immune response
- Altered circulation (lymph, blood)
- Presence of favorable conditions for infection (see Etiologic and Contributing Factors)

Injury, Potential for

DEFINITION

Potential for Injury: The state in which an individual is at risk for injury because of a perceptual or physiological deficit, a lack of awareness, or maturational age.

ETIOLOGICAL AND CONTRIBUTING FACTORS

Pathophysiological

- Altered cerebral circulatory function
  - Tissue hypoxia
  - Post-trauma
  - Vertigo
  - Syncope
  - Confusion
- Altered mobility
  - Unsteady gait
  - Loss of limb
- Impaired sensory function
  - Vision
  - Hearing
  - Thermal/touch
  - Smell
- Pain
- Fatigue

Situational

Faulty judgment
Drugs
Alcohol
Poisons (plants, toxic chemicals)
Household hazards
- Unsafe walkways
- Unsafe toys
- Faulty electric wires
- Improperly stored poisons

Automotive hazards
- Lack of use of seat belts or child seats
- Mechanically unsafe vehicle

Fire hazards
- Smoking in bed
- Gas leaks
- Improperly stored petroleum products

Unfamiliar setting (hospital, nursing home)
Improper footwear
Inattentive caretaker
Improper use of aids (crutches, canes, walkers, wheelchairs)

Maturational

Infant/child
- Suffocation hazards (improper crib, pillow in crib, plastic bags, unattended in water [bath, pool])
- Improper use of bicycles, kitchen utensils/appliances, sports equipment, lawn equipment
- Poison (plants, cleaning agents, medications)
- Fire (matches, fireplace, stove)

Adolescent: Automobile, bicycle, alcohol, drugs
Adult: Automobile, alcohol
Elderly: Motor and sensory deficits, medication (accidental overdose)

DEFINING CHARACTERISTICS

Evidence of environmental hazards
Lack of knowledge of environmental hazards
Lack of knowledge of safety precautions
History of accidents
Impaired mobility
Sensory deficits

Knowledge Deficit: (specify)

DEFINITION

Knowledge Deficit: The state in which the individual experiences a deficiency in cognitive knowledge or psychomotor skills that alters or may alter health maintenance.

ETIOLOGICAL AND CONTRIBUTING FACTORS

A variety of factors can produce knowledge deficits. Some common causes are listed below.

Pathophysiological

Any existing or new medical condition

Situational

- Language differences
- Prescribed treatments (new, complex)
- Diagnostic tests
- Surgical procedures
- Medications
- Pregnancy
- Personal characteristics
  - Lack of motivation
  - Denial of situation
  - Ineffective coping patterns (*e.g.*, anxiety, depression)

Maturational

- Children
  - Sexuality and sexual development
  - Safety hazards
  - Substance abuse
  - Nutrition
- Adolescents
  - Same as children
  - Automobile safety practices
  - Substance abuse (alcohol, drugs, tobacco)
  - Health maintenance practices
- Adults
  - Parenthood
  - Safety practices

Sexual function

Elderly

Effects of aging

Health maintenance practices

Sensory deficits

DEFINING CHARACTERISTICS

Verbalizes a deficiency in knowledge or skill
Expresses "inaccurate" perception of health status
Does not correctly perform a desired or prescribed health behavior because of inadequate knowledge
Does not comply (noncompliance) with prescribed health behavior
Exhibits or expresses psychological alteration (*e.g.*, anxiety, depression) resulting from misinformation or lack of information

Mobility, Impaired Physical

DEFINITION

Impaired Physical Mobility: A state in which the individual experiences, or is at risk of experiencing, limitation of physical movement.

ETIOLOGICAL AND CONTRIBUTING FACTORS

Pathophysiological

Neuromuscular impairment
- Autoimmune alterations (multiple sclerosis, arthritis)
- Nervous system diseases (parkinsonism, myasthenia gravis)
- Muscular dystrophy
- Partial or total paralysis (spinal cord injury, stroke)
- Central nervous system (CNS) tumor
- Increased intracranial pressure
- Sensory deficits

Musculoskeletal impairment
- Spasms
- Flaccidity, atrophy, weakness

Connective tissue disease (systemic lupus erythematosus)
Edema (increased synovial fluid)

Situational

Trauma or surgical procedures
Nonfunctioning or missing limbs (fractures, amputations)
External devices (casts or splints, braces, IV tubing)
Pain
Bedrest

Maturational

Elderly: Decreased motor agility, muscle weakness

DEFINING CHARACTERISTICS

Inability to move purposefully within the environment; including bed mobility, transfers, and ambulation
Inability to move because of imposed restrictions (*e.g.*, bed rest and mechanical and medical protocols)
Range-of-motion limitations
Limited muscle strength or control
Impaired coordination
Impaired perception of position or presence of body parts

Noncompliance

DEFINITION

Noncompliance: The state in which the individual demonstrates personal behavior that deviates from health-related advice given by health care professionals.*

* The use of the nursing diagnosis *Noncompliance* describes the individual who desires to comply, but the presence of certain factors prevents him from doing so. The nurse must attempt to reduce or eliminate these factors for the interventions to be successful. However, the nurse is cautioned against using the diagnosis of noncompliance to describe an individual who has made an informed autonomous decision not to comply.

ETIOLOGICAL AND CONTRIBUTING FACTORS

Many factors in an individual's life can contribute to noncompliance. Some common ones are listed below.

Situational

Side-effects of therapy
Impaired ability to perform tasks (poor memory, motor and sensory deficits)
Previous unsuccessful experience with advised regimen
Increasing amount of disease-related symptoms despite adherence to advised regimen
Concurrent illness of family member
Impersonal aspects of the referral process
Nontherapeutic environment
Inclement weather that prevents person from keeping appointment
Complex, prolonged, or unsupervised therapy
Expensive therapy
Nonsupportive family
Nontherapeutic relationship between client and nurse
Knowledge deficit
Lack of autonomy in health-seeking behavior
Health beliefs that run counter to professional advice
Poor self-esteem
Disturbance in body image

DEFINING CHARACTERISTICS

Verbalization of noncompliance or nonparticipation

Associated Defining Characteristics

Missed appointments
Partially used or unused medications
Persistence of symptoms*
Progression of disease process*
Occurrence of undesired outcomes* (postoperative morbidity, pregnancy, obesity, addiction, regression during rehabilitation)

* When these characteristics are considered to be the result of noncompliance, one is assuming that the therapy prescribed has been proven to be effective and is appropriate.

Nutrition, Alterations in: Less Than Body Requirements

DEFINITION

Alteration in Nutrition: Less Than Body Requirements: The state in which an individual experiences, or is at risk of experiencing, reduced weight related to inadequate intake of nutrients.*

ETIOLOGICAL AND CONTRIBUTING FACTORS

Pathophysiological

- Hyperanabolic/catabolic states
  - Burns (postacute phase)
  - Infection
  - Cancer
  - Trauma
- Chemical dependence
- Dysphagia
  - Cerebrovascular accident
  - Amyotrophic lateral sclerosis
  - Muscular dystrophy
- Absorptive disorders
  - Crohn's disease
  - Intestinal obstruction (ileus)
- Stomatitis
  - Medications or chemotherapy

Situational

- Anorexia
- Depression
- Stress
- Social isolation
- Nausea and vomiting
- Allergy
- Radiation therapy

* This diagnostic category should not be used with individuals who are unable to ingest or absorb nutrients.

Parasites
Inability to procure food (physical limitations, financial or transportation problems)
Lack of knowledge of adequate nutrition
Crash or fad diet
Inability to chew (wired jaw, damaged or missing teeth, ill-fitting dentures)

Maturational

Infants/children: Congenital anomalies, growth spurts
Adolescent: Anorexia nervosa (post-acute phase)
Elderly: Altered sense of taste

DEFINING CHARACTERISTICS

Weight 10% to 20% below ideal for height and frame
Triceps skin fold, mid-arm circumference, and mid-arm muscle circumference less than 60% of the standard measurement
Reported inadequate food intake less than minimum daily requirement (MDR)
Actual or potential metabolic needs in excess of intake

Associated Defining Characteristics

(severe deficiencies)

Tachycardia on minimal exercise and bradycardia at rest
Muscle weakness and tenderness
Mental irritability or confusion
Decreased serum albumin
Decreased serum transferrin or iron-binding capacity
Decreased lymphocyte count

Nutrition, Alterations in: More Than Body Requirements

DEFINITION

Alterations in Nutrition: More Than Body Requirements: The state in which the individual experiences, or is at risk of experiencing, weight gain related to an intake in excess of metabolic requirements.*

ETIOLOGICAL AND CONTRIBUTING FACTORS

Pathophysiological

Altered satiety patterns
Decreased sense of taste and smell

Situational

Anxiety, depression, stress, loneliness, boredom, guilt
Sedentary life-style
Pregnancy (at risk to gain more than 25–30 pounds)
Lack of basic nutritional knowledge
Ethnic or cultural values and expectations that emphasize hearty eating and a hefty body weight

Maturational

Adult/elderly: Decreased activity patterns; decreased metabolic needs

DEFINING CHARACTERISTICS

Overweight (weight 10% over ideal for height and frame)
Obese (weight 20% or more over ideal for height and frame)
Triceps skin fold greater than 15 mm in men and 25 mm in women
Reported undesirable eating patterns
Intake in excess of metabolic requirements
Sedentary activity patterns

Oral Mucous Membrane, Alterations in

DEFINITION

Alterations in Oral Mucous Membrane: The state in which an individual experiences, or is at risk of experiencing, disruptions in the oral cavity.

* The individual *at risk* for weight gain can be described by the label Alteration in Nutrition: Potential for More Than Body Requirements.

ETIOLOGICAL AND CONTRIBUTING FACTORS

Pathophysiological

Diabetes mellitus
Oral cancer
Periodontal disease
Infection
- Herpes simplex
- Gingivitis

Situational

Chemical trauma
- Acidic foods
- Drugs
- Noxious agents
- Alcohol
- Tobacco

Mechanical trauma
- Broken or jagged teeth
- Ill-fitting dentures
- Braces
- Endotracheal tube
- Nasogastric tube

Radiation to head or neck
Malnutrition
Dehydration
Mouth breathing
NPO > 24 hours
Inadequate oral hygiene
Lack of knowledge
Fractured mandible
Prolonged use of steroids or other immunosuppressives
Antineoplastic drugs

DEFINING CHARACTERISTICS

Coated tongue
Xerostomia (dry mouth)
Stomatitis
Oral tumors
Oral lesions
Leukoplakia
Edema
Hemorrhagic gingivitis
Purulent drainage

Parenting, Alterations in

DEFINITION

Alterations in Parenting: The state in which one or more individuals experience a real or potential inability to provide a constructive environment that nurtures the growth and development of his/her/their child (children).*

ETIOLOGICAL AND CONTRIBUTING FACTORS

Individuals or families who may be at high risk for developing or experiencing parenting difficulties include the following:

Parent(s)
- Single
- Adolescent
- Abusive
- Emotionally disturbed
- Alcoholic
- Addicted to drugs
- Terminally ill
- Acutely disabled
- Accident victim

Child
- Of unwanted pregnancy
- Of undesired sex
- With undesired characteristics
- Physically handicapped
- Mentally handicapped
- Hyperactive
- Terminally ill
- Rebellious

Situational

Separation from nuclear family
Lack of extended family
Lack of knowledge
Economic problems
- Inflation
- Unemployment

Relationship problems
- Marital discord
- Divorce
- Separation
- Step-parents
- Live-in boy/girl friend
- Relocation

Change in family unit
- New child
- Relative moves in

Other

History of ineffective relationships with own parents
Parental history of abusive relationship with parents
Unrealistic expectations of child by parent
Unrealistic expectations of self by parent
Unrealistic expectations of parent by child

* A family's ability to function is at a high risk for developing problems when the child or parent has a condition that increases the stress of the family unit.

Unmet psychosocial needs of child by parent
Unmet psychosocial needs of parent by child

DEFINING CHARACTERISTICS

Lack of parental attachment behavior
Diminished or inappropriate visual, tactile, or auditory stimulation of infant
Frequent verbalization of dissatisfaction or disappointment with infant/child
Verbalization of frustration of role
Verbalization of perceived or actual inadequacy
Evidence of abuse or neglect of child
Growth and development lag in infant/child
Inappropriate parenting behaviors

Powerlessness

DEFINITION

Powerlessness: The state in which an individual perceives a lack of personal control over certain events or situations.*

ETIOLOGICAL AND CONTRIBUTING FACTORS

Pathophysiological

Any disease process, acute or chronic, can cause or contribute to powerlessness. Some common sources are

Inability to communicate (CVA, Guillain-Barré, intubation)

* Most individuals are subject to feelings of powerlessness in varying degrees in various situations. This diagnostic category can be used to describe individuals who respond to loss of control with apathy, anger, or depression.

Inability to perform activities of daily living (CVA, cervical trauma, myocardial infarction, pain)
Inability to perform role responsibilities (surgery, trauma, arthritis)
Progressive debilitating disease (multiple sclerosis, terminal cancer)

Situational

Lack of knowledge
Personal characteristics that highly value control (*e.g.,* internal locus of control)
Hospital or institutional limitations
- Some control relinquished to others
- No privacy
- Altered personal territory
- Not consulted regarding decisions
- Social isolation
- Lack of explanations from caregivers

Social displacement
Relocation
Insufficient finances
Sexual harassment

Maturational

Adolescent: Dependence on peer group, independence from family
Young adult: Marriage, pregnancy, parenthood
Adult: Adolescent children, physical signs of aging, career pressures
Elderly: Sensory deficits, motor deficits, losses (money, significant others)

DEFINING CHARACTERISTICS

Expresses dissatisfaction over inability to control situation (*e.g.,* illness, prognosis, care, recovery rate)
Refuses or is reluctant to participate in decision making

Associated defining characteristics

Apathy
Aggressive behavior
Violent behavior
Anxiety
Uneasiness
Resignation
Acting-out behavior
Depression

Rape Trauma Syndrome

DEFINITION

Rape trauma syndrome: A state in which the individual experiences a forced, violent sexual assault (vaginal or anal penetration) against his or her will and without his or her consent. The trauma syndrome that develops from this attack or attempted attack includes an acute phase of disorganization of the victim and family's life-style and a long-term process of reorganization of life-style.*

DEFINING CHARACTERISTICS

If the victim is a child, parent(s) may experience similar responses

Acute Phase

- Somatic responses
  - Gastrointestinal irritability (nausea, vomiting, anorexia)
  - Genitourinary discomfort (pain, pruritus)
  - Skeletal muscle tension (spasms, pain)
- Psychological responses
  - Denial
  - Emotional shock
  - Anger
  - Fear of being alone or that the rapist will return (a child victim will fear punishment, repercussions, abandonment, and/or rejection)
  - Guilt
  - Panic on seeing assailant or scene of the attack
- Sexual responses
  - Mistrust of men (if victim is a woman)
  - Change in sexual behavior

* Holmstrom L, Burgess AW: Development of diagnostic categories: Sexual traumas. Am J Nurs 75:1288–1291, 1975

Long-term Phase

Any response of the acute phase may continue if resolution does not occur.

- Psychological responses
  - Phobias
  - Nightmares or sleep disturbances
  - Anxiety
  - Depression

Respiratory Function, Alterations in

Ineffective Airway Clearance
Ineffective Breathing Patterns
Impaired Gas Exchange

DEFINITION

*Alterations in Respiratory Function (AIRF):** The state in which the individual experiences a real or potential threat to the passage of air through the respiratory tract, and to the exchange of gases (O_2–CO_2) between the lungs and the vascular system.

* This diagnostic category has been added by the author to describe a state in which the entire respiratory system is affected, not just isolated areas such as airway clearance or gas exchange. Smoking, allergy, and immobility are examples of factors that affect the entire system and therefore make it incorrect to say *Impaired Gas Exchange Related to Immobility* because immobility also affects airway clearance and breathing patterns. The three diagnoses *Ineffective Airway Clearance, Ineffective Breathing Patterns,* and *Impaired Gas Exchange* can be used when the contributing factor affects a specific respiratory function. The nurse is cautioned not to use this diagnostic category to describe acute respiratory disorders, which are the primary responsibility of medicine and nursing.

ETIOLOGICAL AND CONTRIBUTING FACTORS

The codes IGE (Impaired Gas Exchange), IAC (Ineffective Airway Clearance), and IBP (Ineffective Breathing Patterns) are used to indicate factors specific to that diagnosis. Factors without a code relate to all four diagnostic categories.

Pathophysiological

- Excessive or thick secretions (IAC, IGE)
- Infection (IAC, IGE)
- Neuromuscular impairment
  - Diseases of the nervous system (*e.g.*, Guillain-Barré syndrome, multiple sclerosis, myasthenia gravis)
  - CNS depression
  - CVA (stroke)
- Loss of lung elasticity
  - COPD (chronic bronchitis, asthma)
  - Aging process
- Decreased lung compliance
- Loss of functioning lung tissue (IGE)
  - Emphysema
  - Atelectasis
  - Tumor
  - Surgery
- Allergic response
- Hypertrophy or edema of upper airway structures—tonsils, adenoids, sinuses (IAC)

Situational

- Surgery or trauma
- Pain, fear, anxiety
- Fatigue
- Mechanical obstruction (IAC, IGE)
- Improper positioning (IAC)
- Altered anatomic structure (IAC, IGE)
  - Tracheostomy
  - Congenital deformity
- Medications (narcotics, sedatives, analgesics)
- Anesthesia, general or spinal (IAC, IBP)
- Aspiration
- Extreme high or low humidity (IAC, IGE)
- Smoking
- Suppressed cough reflex (IAC)
- Bedrest or immobility

Severe nonrelieved cough (IAC, IBP)
Exercise intolerance
Decreased oxygen in the inspired air (IGE)
Mouth breathing (IAC, IBP)
Perception/cognitive impairment (IAC)

Maturational

Neonate: Complicated delivery, prematurity, cesarian birth, low birth weight
Infant/child: Asthma or allergies, increased emesis (aspiration), croup, cystic fibrosis, small airway
Elderly: Decreased surfactant in the lungs, decreased elasticity of the lungs, immobility, slowing of reflexes

DEFINING CHARACTERISTICS

Asymmetrical expansion of chest
Changes in rate of respiration (from baseline)
Changes in depth of respiration (from baseline)
Changes in pattern of respiration (from baseline)
Cyanosis
Rales, rhonchi, fremitus, heaves, wheezes
Alterations in blood gases
Cough
Report of dyspnea
Report of orthopnea
Nasal flaring
Anxiety or restlessness
See also Ineffective Breathing Patterns, Impaired Gas Exchange, Ineffective Airway Clearance

Ineffective Airway Clearance

DEFINITION

Ineffective Airway Clearance: The state in which the individual experiences a real or potential threat to the passage of air through the respiratory tract related to partial or complete airway obstruction.

DEFINING CHARACTERISTICS

Abnormal respiratory rate, rhythm, or depth
Nasal flaring
Ineffective cough
Dyspnea, shortness of breath
Cyanosis, pallor, diaphoresis
Asymmetrical expansion of the chest
Inability to remove secretions
Abnormal breath sounds

Ineffective Breathing Patterns

DEFINITION

Ineffective Breathing Patterns: The state in which the individual experiences an actual or potential loss of adequate ventilation related to an altered breathing pattern.

ETIOLOGICAL AND CONTRIBUTING FACTORS

See Alterations in Respiratory Function

DEFINING CHARACTERISTICS

Orthopnea
Tachypnea, hyperpnea, hyperventilation
Arrhythmic respirations
Splinted/guarded respirations

Impaired Gas Exchange

DEFINITION

Impaired Gas Exchange: The state in which the individual experiences an actual or potential decreased passage of gases (oxygen and carbon dioxide) between the alveoli of the lungs and the vascular system.

ETIOLOGICAL AND CONTRIBUTING FACTORS

See Alterations in Respiratory Function

DEFINING CHARACTERISTICS

Tendency to assume three-point position (sitting, one hand on each knee, bending forward)
Pursed-lip breathing with prolonged expiratory phase
Increased anteroposterior chest diameter, if chronic
Lethargy and fatigue
Increased pulmonary vascular resistance (increased pulmonary artery/right ventricular pressure)
Decreased gastric motility, prolonged gastric emptying
Decreased oxygen content, decreased oxygen saturation, increased pCO_2, as measured by blood gases
Cyanosis

Self-Care Deficit

DEFINITION

Self-Care Deficit: The state in which the individual experiences an impaired motor function or cognitive function, causing a decreased ability to feed, bathe, dress, or toilet oneself.

ETIOLOGICAL AND CONTRIBUTING FACTORS

Pathophysiological

Neuromuscular impairment
- Autoimmune alterations (arthritis, multiple sclerosis)
- Metabolic and endocrine alterations (diabetes mellitus, hypothyroidism)
- Nervous system disorders (parkinsonism, myasthenia gravis, muscular dystrophy)
- Lack of coordination
- Spasticity or flaccidity

- Muscular weakness
- Partial or total paralysis (spinal cord injury, stroke)
- Central nervous system (CNS) tumors
- Increased intracranial pressure

Musculoskeletal disorders

- Atrophy
- Muscle contractures
- Connective tissue diseases (systemic lupus erythematosus)
- Edema (increased synovial fluid)

Visual disorders

- Glaucoma
- Cataracts
- Diabetic/hypertensive retinopathy
- Ocular histoplasmosis
- Cranial nerve neuropathy
- Visual field cuts

Situational

Immobility

Trauma or surgical procedures

- Fractures
- Tracheotomy
- Gastrostomy
- Jejunostomy
- Ileostomy
- Colostomy

Nonfunctioning or missing limbs

External devices (casts or splints, braces, IV equipment)

Maturational

Elderly: Decreased visual and motor ability, muscle weakness

DEFINING CHARACTERISTICS

Self-feeding deficits

- Is unable to cut food
- Is unable to bring food to mouth

Self-bathing deficit (includes washing entire body, combing hair, brushing teeth, attending to skin and nail care, and applying makeup)

- Is unwilling or unable to
  - Wash body or body parts
  - Obtain a water source
  - Regulate temperature or water flow

Self-dressing deficit (including donning regular or special clothing, not nightclothes)
- Has impaired ability to
  - Groom self satisfactorily
  - Put on or take off clothing
  - Fasten clothing
  - Obtain or replace articles of clothing

Self-toileting deficit
- Is unable or unwilling to
  - Get to the toilet or commode
  - Transfer to and from toilet or commode
  - Handle clothing
  - Carry out proper hygiene
  - Flush toilet or empty commode

Self-Concept, Disturbance in

DEFINITION

Disturbance in Self-Concept: The state in which the individual experiences, or is at risk of experiencing, a negative state of change about the way he feels, thinks, or views himself. It may include a change in body image, self-esteem, role performance, or personal identity.

ETIOLOGICAL AND CONTRIBUTING FACTORS

A disturbance in self-concept can occur as a response to a variety of health problems, situations, and conflicts. Some common sources follow.

Pathophysiological

- Loss of body part(s)
- Loss of body function(s)
- Severe trauma

Situational

- Divorce, separation from or death of a significant other
- Loss of job or ability to work

Hospitalization; chronic or terminal illness
Pain
Surgery
Obesity
Pregnancy
Immobility or loss of function
Need for nursing home placement

Maturational

Infant and pre-school: Deprivation
Young adult: Peer pressure, puberty
Middle aged: Signs of aging (graying or loss of hair), reduced hormonal levels (menopause)
Elderly: Losses (people, function, financial, retirement)

Other

Women's movement
Sexual revolution

DEFINING CHARACTERISTICS

Because a disturbance in self-concept may include a change in any one or any combination of its four component parts (body image, self-esteem, role performance, personal identity), and because the nature of the change causing the alteration can be so varied, there is no "typical" response to this diagnosis. Reactions may include

Refusal to touch or look at a body part
Refusal to look into a mirror
Unwillingness to discuss a limitation, deformity, or disfigurement
Refusal to accept rehabilitation efforts
Inappropriate attempts to direct own treatment
Denial of the existence of a deformity or disfigurement
Increasing dependence on others
Signs of grieving: weeping, despair, anger
Refusal to participate in own care or take responsibility for self-care (self-neglect)
Self-destructive behavior (alcohol, drug abuse)
Displaying hostility toward the healthy
Withdrawal from social contacts
Changing usual patterns of responsibility

Showing change in ability to estimate relationship of body to environment

Sensory-Perceptual Alterations

DEFINITION

Sensory-Perceptual Alterations: A state in which the individual experiences, or is at risk of experiencing, a change in the amount, pattern, or interpretation of incoming stimuli.*

ETIOLOGICAL AND CONTRIBUTING FACTORS

Many factors in an individual's life can contribute to sensory-perceptual alterations. Some common factors are listed below.

Pathophysiological

Sensory organ alterations (visual, gustatory, hearing, olfactory, and tactile deficits)

Neurologic alterations
- Cerebrovascular accident (CVA)
- Neuropathies
- Encephalitis meningitis

Metabolic alterations
- Fluid and electrolyte imbalance
- Acidosis
- Alkalosis
- Elevated blood urea nitrogen (BUN)

* This diagnostic category differs from the diagnostic category *Alterations in Thought Processes,* which also describes an individual with cognitive alterations; however, those latter alterations are the results of personality and mental disorders, while these alterations are the results of physiological, sensory, motor, or environmental disruptions. This individual is experiencing a change in usual response to stimuli.

Impaired oxygen transport
- Cerebral
- Cardiac
- Respiratory
- Anemia

Musculoskeletal changes
- Paraplegia
- Quadriplegia
- Amputation

Situational

Medications (sedatives, tranquilizers)
Surgery (glaucoma, cataract, detached retina)
Social isolation (terminal or infectious patient)
Physical isolation (reverse isolation, communicable disease, prison)
Radiation therapy
Immobility
Pain
Stress
Environment (noise pollution)
Mobility restrictions (bedrest, traction, casts, Stryker frame, Circoelectric bed)
Biorhythm alterations (travel, shift-work, hospitalization, special care units [cardiac, trauma, burn])
Substance abuse (alcohol, drugs)
Different culture or language

Maturational

Infant/child: Maternal deprivation, excessive stimulation
Elderly: Hearing or vision loss, gustatory/olfactory deficits, decreased potential for tactile stimulation, isolation, custodial care

DEFINING CHARACTERISTICS

Disoriented in time or place
Disoriented about people
Altered ability to problem-solve
Altered behavior or communication pattern
Sleep pattern disturbances
Restlessness
Reports auditory or visual hallucinations
Fear
Anxiety
Apathy

Sexual Dysfunction

DEFINITION

Sexual Dysfunction: The state in which an individual experiences, or is at risk of experiencing, a change in sexual health or sexual function that is viewed as unrewarding or inadequate.

ETIOLOGICAL AND CONTRIBUTING FACTORS

An alteration in sexual patterns can occur as a response to a variety of health problems, situations, and conflicts. Some common sources are indicated below.

Pathophysiological

- Endocrine
  - Diabetes mellitus
  - Decreased hormone production
  - Myxedema
  - Hyperthyroidism
  - Addison's disease
  - Acromegaly
- Genitourinary
  - Chronic renal failure
  - Premature or retarded ejaculation
  - Priapism
  - Chronic vaginal infection
  - Decreased vaginal lubrication
  - Vaginismus
  - Altered structures
  - Venereal disease
- Neuromuscular and skeletal
  - Arthritis
  - Multiple sclerosis
  - Amyotrophic lateral sclerosis
  - Disturbances of nerve supply to brain, spinal cord, sensory nerves, and autonomic nerves
- Cardiorespiratory
  - Myocardial infarction
  - Congestive heart failure
  - Peripheral vascular disorders
  - Chronic respiratory disorders

Cancer
Liver disease

Psychological

Fear of failure
Fear of pregnancy
Depression
Anxiety
Guilt
Vulnerability

Situational

Partner
- Unwilling
- Uninformed
- Abusive
- Not available
- Separated
- Divorced

Environment
- Unfamiliar
- No privacy
- Hospital

Stressors
- Job problems
- Financial worries
- Conflicting values
- Religious conflict

Lack of knowledge
Fatigue
Obesity
Pain
Alcohol ingestion
Medications
Radiation treatment
Altered self-concept from change in appearance (trauma, radical surgery)

Maturational

Ineffective role models
Negative sexual teaching
Absence of sexual teaching
Aging (separation, isolation)

DEFINING CHARACTERISTICS

Verbalization of problem
Dissatisfaction with sex role (perceived or actual)
Reports limitations on sexual performance imposed by disease or therapy
Fears future limitations on sexual performance
Misinformed about sexuality

Lacks knowledge about sexuality and sexual function
Value conflicts involving sexual expression (cultural, religious)
Reports sexual dissatisfaction or decreased libido
Altered relationship with significant other

Skin Integrity, Impairment of

DEFINITION

Impairment of Skin Integrity: A state in which the individual's skin is altered or is at risk of becoming altered.

ETIOLOGICAL AND CONTRIBUTING FACTORS

Pathophysiological

Autoimmune alterations
- Lupus erythematosus
- Scleroderma

Metabolic and endocrine alterations
- Diabetes mellitus
- Hepatitis
- Cirrhosis
- Renal failure
- Jaundice
- Cancer

Nutritional alterations
- Obesity
- Dehydration
- Edema
- Emaciation

Impaired oxygen transport
- Peripheral vascular alterations
- Arteriosclerosis
- Anemia
- Cardiopulmonary disorders

Medications (steroid therapy)

Psoriasis

Infections
- Bacterial (impetigo, folliculitis, cellulitis)
- Viral (herpes zoster [shingles], herpes simplex)
- Fungal (ringworm [dermatophytosis], athlete's foot, vaginitis)

Situational

Chemical
- Radiation
- Hyperthermia
- Excretions
- Secretions

Environmental
- Humidity
- Parasites
- Bites (insect, animal)
- Contact dermatitis (poison plants—ivy, sumac)

Immobility
- Imposed
- Related to pain, fatigue, motivation, sedation

Stress
Pregnancy
Allergy (drug, food)
Surgery

Maturational

Infants and children: Diaper rash, childhood diseases (chicken pox)
Elderly: Dryness, thin skin

DEFINING CHARACTERISTICS

Denuded skin
Erythema
Lesions (primary, secondary)
Pruritus
Disruptions of skin layer (incision, pressure sores, stomas, fistulas, burns

---

Sleep Pattern Disturbance

DEFINITION

Sleep Pattern Disturbance. The state in which the individual experiences, or is at risk of experiencing, a change in the quantity or quality of his rest pattern as related to his biologic and emotional needs.

ETIOLOGICAL AND CONTRIBUTING FACTORS

Many factors in an individual's life can contribute to sleep pattern disturbances. Some common factors are listed below.

Pathophysiological

- Impaired oxygen transport
  - Angina
  - Peripheral arteriosclerosis
  - Respiratory disorders
  - Circulatory disorders
- Impaired elimination (bowel or bladder)
  - Diarrhea
  - Constipation
  - Incontinence
  - Retention
  - Dysuria
  - Frequency
- Impaired metabolism
  - Hyperthyroidism
  - Gastric ulcers
  - Hepatic disorders

Situational

- Immobility (imposed by casts, traction)
- Lack of exercise
- Pain
- Anxiety response
- Pregnancy
- Life-style disruptions
  - Occupational
  - Emotional
  - Social
  - Sexual
  - Financial
- Environmental changes
  - Hospitalization (noise, disturbing roommate, fear)
  - Travel
- Medications
  - Tranquilizers
  - Sedatives
  - Hypnotics
  - Antidepressants
  - Antihypertensives
  - Amphetamines
  - Steroids
  - Soporifics
  - Monoamine (MAO) inhibitors
  - Anesthetics
  - Barbiturates

Maturational

- Neonates: Hypoxia
- Infants and children: Nightmares, fears
- Adults: Parenthood
- Elderly: Chronic illness, depression

DEFINING CHARACTERISTICS

Adults

Difficulty falling asleep or remaining asleep
Fatigue on awakening or during the day
Dozing during the day
Agitation
Mood alterations

Children

Sleep disturbances in children are frequently related to fear, enuresis, or inconsistent responses of parents to child's requests for changes in sleep rules, such as requests to stay up late.

Reluctance to retire
Frequent awakening during the night
Desire to sleep with parents

Social Interactions, Impaired

DEFINITION

Impaired Social Interactions: The state in which the individual experiences, or is at risk of experiencing, negative, insufficient, or unsatisfactory responses (outcomes) from interactions.

ETIOLOGICAL AND CONTRIBUTING FACTORS

Pathophysiological

Loss of body part
Loss of body function
Terminal disease
Hearing deficits
Visual deficits

Situational

Severe trauma
Obesity

Disfigurement/disability
Depression
Anxiety
Language/cultural barriers
Altered self-concept
Substance use disorder (alcohol, drugs)

Emotional and Behavioral Disorders

Somatoform
Paranoid
Bipolar
Schizophrenic
Adjustment/anxiety
Affective personality

Maturational

Child/adolescent
  Speech impediments
  Altered appearance (braces, acne)

Social Isolation

DEFINITION

Social Isolation: The state in which the individual experiences a need or desire for contact with others but is unable to make that contact.*

ETIOLOGICAL AND CONTRIBUTING FACTORS

A state of social isolation can result from a variety of situations and health problems that are related to a loss of established relationships or to a failure to generate these relationships. Some common sources follow.

* Social isolation is a negative state of aloneness. It is a subjective state that exists whenever a person says it does and is perceived as imposed by others. Social isolation is *not* the voluntary solitude that is necessary for personal renewal, nor is it the creative aloneness of the artist or the loneliness (and possible suffering) that one may experience as a result of seeking individualism and independence (*e.g.*, moving to a new city, going away to college).

Situational

Death of a significant other
Divorce
Extreme poverty
Hospitalization or terminal illness (dying process)
Moving to another culture (*e.g.*, unfamiliar language)
Drug or alcohol addiction
Obesity
Cancer (disfiguring surgery of head or neck, superstitions of others)
Physical handicaps (paraplegia, amputation, arthritis, hemiplegia)
Emotional handicaps (extreme anxiety, depression, paranoia, phobias)
Homosexuality
Loss of usual means of transportation
Incontinence (embarrassment, odor)

Maturational

Elderly: Sensory losses, motor losses, loss of significant others

DEFINING CHARACTERISTICS

Because social isolation is a subjective state, all inferences made regarding a person's feelings of aloneness must be validated. Because the causes vary and people show their aloneness in different ways, there are no absolute cues to this diagnosis.

Possible Subjective Reactions

Expressed feelings of unexplained dread or abandonment
Desire for more family or nurse contact
Time passing slowly ("Mondays are so long for me")

Associated Characteristics

Inability to concentrate and make decisions
Feelings of uselessness
Doubts about ability to survive

Behavior Changes

Increased irritability or restlessness
Underactivity (physical or verbal)

Inability to make decisions
Increased signs and symptoms of illness (a change from previous state of good health)
Appearing depressed, anxious, or angry
Postponing important decision-making
Failure to interact with others nearby
Sleep disturbance (too much sleep or insomnia)
Change in eating habits (overeating or anorexia)

Social isolation can result in other problems and responses. These include anxiety, depression, fear, nutritional alterations, and a threatened self-image.

See also *Anxiety, Alterations in Thought Processes, Powerlessness, Ineffective Individual Coping Related to Depression, Fear, Alterations in Nutrition,* and *Disturbance in Self-Concept.*

Spiritual Distress

DEFINITION

Spiritual Distress: The state in which the individual experiences, or is at risk of experiencing, a disturbance in his belief or value system that is his source of strength and hope.

ETIOLOGICAL AND CONTRIBUTING FACTORS

Spiritual distress can occur as a response to a variety of health problems, situations, and conflicts. Some common sources follow.

Pathophysiological

Loss of body part or function
Terminal disease
Debilitating disease

Situational

Death or illness of significant other
Embarrassment at practicing spiritual rituals
Hospital barriers to practicing spiritual rituals
- Isolation
- Intensive care restrictions
- Surgery
- Medications
- Confinement to bed or room
- Trauma
- Dietary restrictions
- Medical procedures (*e.g.*, IVs)

Conflicts to belief system
- Abortion
- Pain
- Divorce
- Surgery or blood transfusion (when prohibited by religion)

Beliefs opposed by family, peers, health care providers

DEFINING CHARACTERISTICS

Experiences a disturbance in belief system
- Questions credibility of belief system
- Is discouraged
- Is unable to practice usual religious rituals
- Has ambivalent feelings (doubts) about beliefs
- Feels a sense of spiritual emptiness

Expresses concern (anger, resentment, fear) about meaning of life, suffering, and death
Requests spiritual assistance for a disturbance in belief system

Thought Processes, Alterations in

DEFINITION

Alterations in Thought Processes: A state in which an individual experiences a disruption in mental activities such as conscious thought, reality orientation, problem solving, judgment, and comprehension related to coping (personality and mental) disorders.*

ETIOLOGICAL AND CONTRIBUTING FACTORS

Pathophysiological

Personality and mental disorders related to alteration in biochemical compounds
Genetic disorder

Situational†

Depression or anxiety
Substance abuse (alcohol, drugs)
Fear of the unknown
Actual loss (of control, routine, income, significant others, familiar object, or surroundings)
Emotional trauma
Rejection or negative appraisal by others
Negative response from others
Isolation

Maturational†

Adolescent: Peer pressure, conflict
Elderly: Isolation

DEFINING CHARACTERISTICS

Disoriented in time, place, or person
Altered abstraction
Distractibility
Memory deficits
Inaccurate interpretation of stimuli

* The diagnosis *Alterations in Thought Processes* describes an individual with cognitive alterations (inaccurate interpretation of the environment) that result from personality and mental disorders. This diagnosis differs from the diagnostic category *Sensory-Perceptual Alterations,* which describes an individual with alterations in the amount, pattern, or interpretation of incoming stimuli that are the result of physiological, sensory, motor, or environmental disruptions, not personality and mental disorders.

† These factors should not be considered causative or contributive unless they are present in an individual with a history of coping disorders.

Tissue Perfusion, Alteration in

DEFINITION

Alteration in Tissue Perfusion: The state in which the individual experiences, or is at risk of experiencing, a decrease in nutrition and respiration at the cellular level due to a decrease in capillary blood supply.*

ETIOLOGICAL AND CONTRIBUTING FACTORS

Physiological

- Cardiovascular disorders
  - Decreased cardiac output
  - Cerebrovascular accident (CVA)
  - Transient ischemic attacks (TIA)
  - Arteriosclerotic vascular disease (ASVD)
  - Atherosclerosis
  - Myocardial infarction (MI)
  - Angina
  - Congestive heart failure
  - Pulmonary edema
  - Varicosities
  - Vasospasm or vasoconstriction
  - Hypertension
- Diabetes mellitus

* The use of this diagnostic category should not include the treatment of decreased tissue perfusion (which is a clinical problem) but should focus on the functional abilities of the individual that are compromised because of decreased tissue perfusion. To represent this relationship, the diagnosis is linked by a colon (:) and not by the phrase "related to." The use of "related to" would label a clinical situation that is more medical than nursing, as with the title "Alteration in Tissue Perfusion: Cardiac, related to Congestive Heart Failure." The nurse can diagnose and treat certain responses to impaired tissue perfusion, in which case the diagnosis can be structured accordingly. For example, *Alteration in Tissue Perfusion: Cerebral: Orthostatic Hypotension or Alteration in Tissue Perfusion: Renal: Fatigue.*

- Hypotension
  - Orthostatic
  - Neurogenic
  - Hypovolemic
  - Drug-induced
- Blood dyscrasias
  - Anemia
  - Polycythemia
  - DIC (disseminating intravascular coagulation)
  - Thrombus
- Renal failure
- Cancer or tumor
- Edema or inflammation
- Septic shock
- Anaphylactic shock
- Hypoglycemia
- Hyperglycemia
- Embolus
- Hemolysis (*e.g.*, transfusion reaction)
- Sickle cell disease

Situational

- Presence of invasive lines (*e.g.*, IVs, Foley catheter [predisposes to thrombi and sepsis])
- Prolonged immobility or bedrest
- Pressure sites (*e.g.*, decubiti, casts, Ace bandages, tourniquets)
- Sudden change from lying or sitting to standing
- Dependent venous pooling (predisposes to thrombus formation)
- Medications (*e.g.*, diuretics, tranquilizers, insulin)
- Anesthesia (causes vasodilation)
- Blood vessel trauma or compression
- Pregnancy or oral contraception (predisposes to thrombus formation)
- Hypothermia (*e.g.*, exposure to cold)
- Obesity (poor circulation)
- Anorexia or malnutrition

Maturational

- Neonate
  - Immature peripheral circulation
  - Rh incompatibility (erythroblastosis fetalis)
  - Hypothermia
- Elderly
  - Venous and arterial capillary fragility
  - Brittle, hard vessels (due to chronic ASVD)

DEFINING CHARACTERISTICS

Peripheral

Loss of motor function
Loss of sensory function
Tissue necrosis (gangrene)
Coolness of skin
Pallor
Cyanosis
Flushing
Claudication (leg pain on walking, relieved by rest)
Decreased pulse quality
Edema
Lack of lanugo hair

Cardiopulmonary

Tachycardia
Tachypnea
Angina (relieved by rest)
Dyspnea

Cerebral

Restlessness
Confusion
Altered thought processes
Memory losses
Altered level of consciousness

Gastrointestinal

Constipation
Nausea or vomiting

Renal

Edema
Decreased urinary output

Urinary Elimination, Alteration in Patterns of

DEFINITION

Alteration in Patterns of Urinary Elimination: The state in which the individual experiences or is at risk of experiencing urinary dysfunction.*

* This diagnostic category pertains to alterations of urine elimination, not urine formation. Nurses can diagnose and treat an alteration in patterns of elimination independently, but they cannot alter polyuria, retention, anuria, and oliguria with independent nursing interventions.

ETIOLOGICAL AND CONTRIBUTING FACTORS

Pathophysiological (except when urine formation is altered)

Congenital urinary tract anomalies
- Strictures
- Hypospadias or epispadias
- Ureterocele
- Bladder-neck contracture
- Megalocystis (large-capacity bladder without tone)

Disorders of the urinary tract
- Infection
- Calculi

Neurogenic disorders or injury
- Cord injury
- Brain tumor
- Cerebrovascular accident
- Multiple sclerosis
- Demyelinating diseases

Prostatic enlargement

Estrogen deficiency
- Vaginitis
- Atrophic urethritis

Situational

Loss of perineal tissue tone
- Scarring of perineal area
- Obesity
- Recent substantial weight loss
- Childbirth
- Aging
- Post prostatectomy

Fecal impaction

Dehydration

Drug therapy
- Antihistamines
- Epinephrine
- Anticholinergics
- Immunosuppressant therapy (chemotherapy)
- Diuretics

Irritation to perineal area
- Sexual activity
- Poor personal hygiene
- Diagnostic instrumentation

Pregnancy

General or spinal anesthesia

Inability to communicate needs

Lack of privacy

Decreased attention to bladder cues
- Sedatives
- Tranquilizers
- Depression
- Confusion

Foley catheters
Stress or fear
Environmental barriers to bathroom
- Distant toilets
- Poor lighting
- Bed too high
- Side rails

Maturational

Child: Small bladder capacity, lack of motivation
Elderly: Motor and sensory losses, loss of muscle tone, inability to communicate needs, depression

DEFINING CHARACTERISTICS

Dysuria
Urgency
Frequency
Hesitancy
Nocturia
Enuresis
Dribbling
Bladder distention
Incontinence

Violence, Potential for

DEFINITION

Potential for Violence: A state in which an individual experiences aggressive behavior that can be directed either at one's self or at others.

ETIOLOGICAL AND CONTRIBUTING FACTORS

Pathophysiological

Temporal lobe epilepsy
Toxic reaction to medication
Toxic response to alcohol or nonprescribed or prescribed drugs
Physical trauma
Physical progressive deterioration (organic brain disease, brain tumor)

Hormonal imbalance
Alteration in biochemical compounds leading to depression or manic depression

Situational

Increase in stressors within a short period of time
Physical immobility
Suicidal behavior
Environmental controls
Perceived threat to self-esteem
Fear of the unknown
Response to catastrophic event
Rage reaction
Misperceived messages from others
Antisocial character
Response to dysfunctional family throughout developmental stages
Dysfunctional communication patterns
Drug or alcohol abuse

DEFINING CHARACTERISTICS

Hostile threats or rage
History of abuse to self or others
Overt aggressive acts
Fear or anxiety
Suspicion of others
Delusions, hallucinations
Agitation, increased motor activity
Rigid body language (clenched fists, clenched jaw)
Depression
Perception of self as worthless or hopeless
Perception of environment as frightening or hostile

Section II

Medical Diagnostic Categories with Possible Associated Nursing Diagnoses

Medical Diagnoses

Cardiovascular/Hematologic/ Peripheral Vascular Disorders

- Cardiac Conditions
  - Angina Pectoris
  - Congestive Heart Failure with Acute Pulmonary Edema
  - Endocarditis, Pericarditis
    - Rheumatic
    - Infectious
  - Myocardial Infarction
- Hematologic Conditions
  - Anemia
    - Aplastic Anemia
    - Pernicious Anemia
  - Disseminated Intravascular Coagulation (DIC)
  - Polycythemia Vera
- Peripheral Vascular Conditions
  - Deep Vein Thrombosis
  - Hypertension
  - Peripheral Vascular Diseases
    - Thromboangiitis Obliterans
    - Stasis Ulcers
  - Varicose Veins
- Surgical Procedures (see section on Surgical Procedures)
  - Abdominal Aortic Aneurysm Resection
  - Arterial Occlusions with Graft, Lower Extremity
    - Femoral
    - Popliteal
    - Aortic
    - Iliac
  - Myocardial Revascularization (Coronary Artery Bypass)
- Diagnostic Studies/Special Therapies (see section on Diagnostic and Therapeutic Procedures)
  - Angioplasty (Percutaneous, Transluminal, Coronary)
  - Anticoagulant Therapy

Arteriogram
Cardiac Catheterization
Hemodynamic Monitoring
Intra-aortic Balloon Pumping
Pacemaker Insertion

Cardiac Conditions

ANGINA PECTORIS

Alterations in Comfort related to chest pain
Fear related to present status and unknown future
Sleep Pattern Disturbances related to treatments and environment
Potential Alterations in Bowel Elimination: Constipation related to bed rest, change in life-style and medications
Activity Intolerance related to fear of recurrent angina
Potential Disturbances in Self-concept related to perceived or actual role changes
Possible Impaired Home Maintenance Management related to angina or fear of angina
Potential Alteration in Family Processes related to impaired ability of person to assume role responsibilities
Potential Sexual Dysfunction related to fear of angina and altered self-concept
Grieving: denial, anger, depression related to actual or perceived losses secondary to cardiac condition
Knowledge Deficit: (specify)
examples:
condition
diet
home activities
medications

CONGESTIVE HEART FAILURE WITH PULMONARY EDEMA

Potential Complications: *
Deep vein thrombosis
Severe hypoxia
Activity Intolerance related to dyspnea and fatigue secondary to decreased cardiac output

* Potential complications are clinical problems, not nursing diagnoses.

Alteration in Nutrition: Less than Body Requirements, related to nausea; anorexia secondary to venous congestion of gastrointestinal tract and fatigue
Alteration in Tissue Perfusion: Peripheral, related to venous congestion
Anxiety related to breathlessness
Fear related to progressive nature of condition
Potential Impaired Home Maintenance related to inability to perform activities of daily living secondary to breathlessness and fatigue
Self Care Deficit: (specify) related to dyspnea and fatigue
Sleep-Rest Dysrhythm related to nocturnal dyspnea and inability to assume usual sleep position
Potential Fluid Volume Excess: Edema related to compensatory kidney mechanisms
Knowledge Deficit: (specify)
examples:
- low-salt diet
- drug therapy (diuretic, digitalis)
- activity program
- signs and symptoms of complications

ENDOCARDITIS, PERICARDITIS
(Rheumatic, Infectious)

See also Corticosteroid Therapy.
If child, see Rheumatic Fever.
Potential Complications:
- *Congestive heart failure*
- *Valve stenosis*
- *Cerebral vascular accident*
- *Emboli (pulmonary, cerebral, renal, spleen, heart)*
- *Cardiac tamponade*

Activity Intolerance related to dyspnea secondary to restriction of heart contraction
Potential Alteration in Respiratory Function related to decreased respiratory depth secondary to pain
Alteration in Comfort: Pain related to friction rub and inflammation process
Knowledge Deficit: (specify)
examples:
- etiology
- prevention
- antibiotic prophylaxis
- signs and symptoms of complications

MYOCARDIAL INFARCTION (Uncomplicated)

Potential Complications:
Dysrhythmias
Cardiac arrest
Cardiogenic shock

Alterations in Comfort: pain related to cardiac tissue ischemia
Fear related to present status and unknown future
Sleep Pattern Disturbances related to treatments and environment
Potential Alterations in Bowel Elimination: Constipation related to bed rest, change in life-style, and medications
Activity Intolerance related to decreased cardiac output and fear of recurrent angina
Potential Disturbances in Self-Concept related to perceived or actual role changes
Possible Impaired Home Maintenance Management related to angina or fear of angina
Potential Alteration in Family Processes related to impaired ability of ill person to assume role responsibilities
Potential Sexual Dysfunction related to fear of angina and altered self-concept
Grieving: denial, anger, and depression related to actual or perceived losses secondary to cardiac condition
Knowledge Deficit: (specify)
examples:
condition
home activities
diet
medications

Hematologic Conditions

ANEMIA

Potential Complications:
Transfusion reaction
Cardiac failure
Iron overload (repeated transfusion)

Activity Intolerance related to fatigue and dyspnea secondary to hypoxia
Potential for Infection related to decreased resistance secondary to abnormal red blood counts (neutropenia, leukopenia)

Potential for Injury: bleeding tendencies related to thrombocytopenia and splenomegaly
Potential Alteration in Oral Mucous Membrane related to gastrointestinal mucosal atrophy
Knowledge Deficit: (specify)
examples:
condition
nutritional requirement
drug therapy

APLASTIC ANEMIA

Potential Complications:
Fatal aplasia
Pancytopenia
Hemorrhage
Hypoxia
Infection

Activity Intolerance related to breathlessness and fatigue secondary to diminished red blood cell count
Potential for Infection related to increased susceptibility secondary to leukopenia
Potential Alteration in Oral Mucous Membrane related to tissue hypoxia and vulnerability
Knowledge Deficit: (specify)
examples:
causes
prevention
signs and symptoms of complications

PERNICIOUS ANEMIA

See also Anemia.

Alteration in Oral Mucous Membrane related to sore red tongue secondary to papillary atrophy and inflammatory changes
Alteration in Bowel Elimination: Diarrhea/Constipation related to gastrointestinal mucosal atrophy
Potential Alteration in Nutrition: Less than Body Requirements, related to anorexia secondary to sore mouth
Knowledge Deficit: (specify)
examples:
chronicity of disease
vitamin-B treatment
familial propensity

DISSEMINATED INTRAVASCULAR COAGULATION (DIC)

See also Underlying Disorders (e.g., *Obstetric, Infections, Burns).*
See also Anticoagulant Therapy.
Potential Complications:
Hemorrhage
Renal failure
Microthrombi (renal, cardiac, pulmonary, cerebral, gastrointestinal)

Anxiety/Fear related to treatments, environment, and risk of death
Alteration in Family Processes related to critical nature of the situation and uncertain prognosis
Potential Sensory Perceptual Alterations related to
examples:
pain
immobility
excessive environmental stimuli
disruption of biorhythms
Knowledge Deficit: (specify)
examples:
causes
treatment

POLYCYTHEMIA VERA

Potential Complications:
Thrombus formation
Hemorrhage
Myelosuppressive agents
Hypertension
Congestive heart failure
Peptic ulcer
Gout

Alteration in Nutrition: Less than Body Requirements related to anorexia, nausea, and vasocongestion
Activity Intolerance related to dyspnea and fatigue secondary to pulmonary congestion and tissue hypoxia
Potential for Infection related to hypoxia secondary to vasocongestion
Knowledge Deficit: (specify)
examples:
fluid requirements
exercise program

signs and symptoms of complications
 thrombi
 congestive heart failure
 hypertension

Peripheral Vascular Conditions

DEEP VEIN THROMBOSIS

See also Anticoagulant Therapy if indicated.
Potential Complications: embolism
Potential Alteration in Bowel Elimination: Constipation related to immobility
Potential Alteration in Respiratory Function related to immobility
Alteration in Tissue Perfusion: Peripheral related to thrombus
Alteration in Comfort: Pain related to impaired circulation (extremities)
Knowledge Deficit: (specify)
 examples:
  prevention of recurrence
  implications of anticoagulant therapy
  exercise program
  foot care

HYPERTENSION

Potential Complications:
 Retinal hemorrhage
 Cerebral vascular accident
 Cerebral hemorrhage
 Renal failure
Potential Noncompliance related to negative side effects of prescribed therapy versus the disbelief that treatment is needed without the presence of symptoms
Potential Sexual Dysfunction related to decreased libido or erectile dysfunction secondary to medication side effects
Knowledge Deficit: (specify)
 examples:
  diet restriction
  medications
  signs of complications
  risk factors (obesity, smoking)
  follow-up care

PERIPHERAL VASCULAR DISEASE

(Thrombangiitis Obliterans; Stasis Ulcers)

Potential Complications:

- *Leg ulcers*
- *Cellulitis*
- *Thrombosis/emboli*

Alteration in Tissue Perfusion: Peripheral related to compromised circulation

Potential Impairment of Skin Integrity related to compromised peripheral circulation

Alteration in Comfort: Pain related to impaired ability of peripheral vessels to supply tissue with oxygen and arterial spasms

Activity Intolerance related to impaired ability of peripheral vessels to supply the needed oxygen for activities

Potential for Injury related to decreased sensation in superficial tissues

Potential for Infection related to trophic changes secondary to prolonged ischemia and malnutrition of tissues

Knowledge Deficit: (specify)

examples:

- condition
- Exercise program
- Prevention of complications
- Signs and symptoms of complications
- risk factors
  - obesity
  - smoking
  - cold
- Foot care
- Diet

VARICOSE VEINS

Potential Complications:

- *Vascular rupture*
- *Hemorrhage*
- *Stasis ulcer*

Alteration in Tissue Perfusion: Peripheral related to varicose veins

Alteration in Comfort: Pain related to edema secondary to venous congestion

Knowledge Deficit: (specify)
examples:
activities of daily living at home
risk factors
follow-up care

Respiratory Disorders

Acute Respiratory Distress Syndrome (ARDS)
Chronic Obstructive Pulmonary Disease (COPD)
Emphysema
Bronchitis
Pleural Effusion
Pneumonia
Pulmonary Embolism
Surgical Procedure (see section on Surgical Procedures)
Thoracic Surgery
Mechanical Ventilation (see index for pages)

ACUTE RESPIRATORY DISTRESS SYNDROME (ARDS)

See also Mechanical Ventilation (under Diagnostic Studies/ Special Therapies).

Potential Complications:
Electrolyte imbalance *Hypoxia*
Of steroid therapy

Anxiety related to implications of condition and critical care setting

Powerlessness related to condition and treatments (ventilator, monitoring)

CHRONIC OBSTRUCTIVE PULMONARY DISEASE—COPD (Emphysema, Bronchitis)

Potential Complications of hypoxemia/hypovolemia:
Electrolyte imbalance *Inadequate cardiac output*
Acid-base imbalance

Ineffective Airway Clearance related to excessive and tenacious mucous secretions

Alteration in Nutrition: Less than Body Requirements, related to dyspnea and loss of appetite
Impaired Gas Exchange related to CO_2 retention and excessive mucous production
Activity Intolerance related to dyspnea and fatigue
Impaired Verbal Communication related to dyspnea
Anxiety related to breathlessness and fear of suffocation
Powerlessness related to loss of control and the restrictions that this condition places on lifestyle
Sleep-Rest Disturbance related to
examples:
- cough
- inability to assume recumbent position
- environment stimuli

Knowledge Deficit
examples:
- condition
- pharmacologic therapy
- nutritional therapy
- prevention of inflection
- rest versus activity
- breathing exercises
- home care (*e.g.* equipment)

PLEURAL EFFUSION

See also Underlying Disorders (congestive heart disease, cirrhosis, malignancy).

Potential Complications:
- *Respiratory failure*
- *Pneumothorax (post-thoracentesis)*
- *Hemothorax*

Activity Intolerance related to dyspnea secondary to hypoxia
Potential Alteration in Nutrition: Less than Body Requirements related to anorexia secondary to pressure on abdominal structures
Alteration in Comfort: Pain and Dyspnea related to accumulation of fluid in pleural space
Self-Care Deficits: (specify) related to fatigue and dyspnea
Alteration in Respiratory Function related to pain

PNEUMONIA

Potential Complications:
- *Hyperthermia*
- *Respiratory insufficiency*
- *Septic shock*
- *Paralytic ileus*

Activity Intolerance related to compromised respiratory
function
Potential Alteration in Oral Mucous Membrane related to
mouth breathing and frequent expectorations
Potential Fluid Volume Deficit related to increased
insensible fluid loss secondary to fever and
hyperventilation
Potential Alteration in Nutrition: Less than Body
Requirements, related to anorexia dyspnea and
abdominal distention secondary to air swallowing
Ineffective Airway Clearance related pain,
tracheobronchial secretions, and exudate
Potential for Inflection to Others related to communicable
nature of the disease
Alteration in Comfort related to hyperthermia, malaise,
and pulmonary pathology
Potential Impairment of Skin Integrity related to
prescribed bed rest
Knowledge Deficit:
examples:
fluid requirements
caloric requirements
medications regime

PULMONARY EMBOLISM

Potential Complications:
Anticoagulant therapy
Potential Impairment of Skin Integrity related to
immobility and prescribed bed rest
Knowledge Deficit: (specify)
examples:
anticoagulant therapy
signs and symptoms of complications

Metabolic/Endocrine Disorders

Addison's Disease
Aldosteronism, Primary
Cirrhosis (Laennec's)
Cushing's Syndrome

Diabetes Mellitus
Hepatitis (Acute, Viral)
Hyperthyroidism
Thyroidtoxicosis
Grave's Disease
Hypothyroidism (Myxedema)
Obesity
Pancreatitis

ADDISON'S DISEASE

Potential Complications:
Addisonian crisis (shock) *Hypoglycemia*
Electrolyte imbalances (sodium, potassium)

Potential Alteration in Nutrition: Less than Body Requirements, related to anorexia and nausea
Potential Fluid Volume Deficit related to excessive loss of sodium and water secondary to polyuria
Activity Intolerance related to fatigue
Alteration in Bowel Elimination: Diarrhea related to increased excretion of sodium and water
Potential Disturbance in Self-Concept related to appearance changes secondary to increased skin pigmentation and decreased axillary and pubic hair (female)
Potential for Injury related to postural hypotension secondary to fluid/electrolyte imbalances
Knowledge Deficit: (specify)
examples:
disease
signs and symptoms of complications
risks for crisis
infection
diarrhea
decreased sodium intake
diaphoresis
overexertion
dietary management
identification (card, tag)
emergency kit
pharmacologic management and titration dose as needed

ALDOSTERONISM, PRIMARY

Potential Complications:

Hypokalemia
Alkalosis
Hypertension
Hypernatremia

Alteration in Comfort: polydipsia related to excessive urine excretion
Potential Fluid Volume Deficit related to excessive urinary excretion
Knowledge Deficit: (specify)
examples:
condition
surgical treatment
corticosteroid therapy

CIRRHOSIS (Laennec's)

See also Substance Abuse if indicated.
Potential Complications:

Hemorrhage
Hypokalemia
Portal systemic encephalopathy
Negative nitrogen balance
Drug toxicity (opiates, short-acting barbiturates, major tranquilizers)
Renal failure
Anemia
Esophageal varices

Alteration in Comfort: Pain related to liver enlargement and ascites
Alteration in Bowel Elimination: Diarrhea related to excessive secretion of fats in stool secondary to liver dysfunction
Potential for Injury related to decreased prothrombin production and synthesis of substances used in blood coagulation
Alteration in Nutrition: Less than Body Requirements, related to anorexia, impaired utilization, and storage of vitamins (A, C, K, D, E)
Activity Intolerance related to fatigue, ascites peripheral edema
Potential Alteration in Respiratory Function related to pressure on diaphragm secondary to ascites
Potential Disturbance in Self-Concept related to appearance changes (jaundice, ascites)

Potential for Infection related to leukopenia secondary to enlarged, overactive spleen and hypoproteinemia
Impairment of Skin Integrity related to pruritis and jaundice secondary to accumulation of bilirubin pigment and bile salts
Fluid Volume Excess related to peripheral edema and ascites secondary to portal hypertension, lowered plasma colloidal osmotic pressure, and sodium retention
Knowledge Deficit: (specify)
examples:
- pharmacologic contraindication
- nutritional requirements
- signs and symptoms of complications
- risks of alcohol

CUSHING'S SYNDROME

Potential Complications:
- *Hypertension*
- *Congestive heart failure*
- *Psychosis*
- *Electrolyte imbalance (sodium, potassium)*

Disturbance in Self-Concept related to physicial changes secondary to disease process (moon face, thinning of hair, truncal obesity, virilism)
Potential for Infection related to excessive protein catabolism and depressed leukocytic phagocytosis secondary to hyperglycemia
Potential for Injury: fractures related to osteoporosis
Activity Intolerance related to fatigue and lassitude
Potential Impairment of Skin Integrity related to loss of tissue, edema, and dryness
Sexual Dysfunction related to loss of libido and cessation of menses (female) secondary to excessive adrenocorticotropic hormone production
Knowledge Deficit: (specify)
examples:
- disease
- diet therapy
  - high protein
  - low CHO
  - low sodium

DIABETES MELLITUS (Adult)

Potential Complications:

- *Hyper- /hypoglycemia*
- *Neuropathies*
- *Vascular (microangiopathy, atherosclerosis)*
- *Infection*
- *Retinopathy*
- *Urinary tract infections*

Potential Impairment of Skin Integrity related to increased susceptibility to fungal infection, pruritis secondary to vascular condition and increased blood sugar

Potential Sexual Dysfunction (male) related to erectile problems secondary to peripheral neuropathy

Potential Sensory Perceptual Alterations: tactile, related to paresthesia secondary to peripheral neuropathies

Potential Sensory Perceptual Alterations: Visual, related to retinopathy

Potential for Injury related to decreased tactile sensation and diminished visual acuity

Alteration in Tissue Perfusion: Peripheral related to decreased neurovascular function secondary to peripheral neuropathies

Potential for Infection related to depleted host defenses and depressed leukocytic phagocytosis secondary to hyperglycemia

Alteration in Nutrition: Greater than Body Requirements related to intake in excess of activity expenditures

Alteration in Nutrition: Less than Body Requirements related to insufficient coverage for caloric requirements to maintain growth and development

Potential Noncompliance related to the complexity of adhering to the prescribed regime

Powerlessness related to the uncertainty of the disease and the development of complications

Knowledge Deficit: (specify)

examples:

- disease
- nutrition (meal planning)
- weight control
- exercise program
- medications
  - type

administration
side effects
foot care
signs and symptoms of complications
record keeping
blood/urine testing
hypoglycemia/hyperglycemia
detection
treatment
community services (support groups)

HEPATITIS (Acute, Viral)

Potential Complications:
Hepatic failure
Coma
Subacute hepatic necrosis
Fulminant hepatitis

Activity Intolerance related to fatigue and weakness secondary to reduced energy metabolism by liver
Potential for Infection to others related to contagious agents
Alteration in Nutrition: Less than Body Requirements related to anorexia, epigastric distress, and nausea
Potential Fluid Volume Deficit related to lack of desire to drink
Impairment of Skin Integrity related to pruritus secondary to bile salt accumulation
Potential for Injury related to reduced prothrombin synthesis and reduced vitamin-K absorption
Alteration in Comfort: Pain related to swelling of inflamed liver
Potential Impaired Social Interactions related to the isolation precautions needed to prevent transmission of the disease
Diversional Activity Deficit related to the monotony of confinement and isolation precautions
Knowledge Deficit: (specify)
examples:
condition
rest requirements
precautions to prevent transmission
nutritional requirements
contraindications
certain medication
alcohol

HYPERTHYROIDISM

(Thyroidtoxicosis, Graves' Disease)

Potential Complications:

Thyroid storm *Cardiac arrhythmias*

Alteration in Nutrition: Less than Body Requirements related to intake less than metabolic needs secondary to excessive metabolic rate

Activity Intolerance related to fatigue and exhaustion secondary to excessive metabolic rate

Alteration in Bowel Elimination: Diarrhea related to increased peristalsis secondary to excessive metabolic rate

Potential for Injury: corneal abrasion related to inability to close eyelids secondary to exophthalmus

Alteration in Comfort related to heat intolerance and profuse diaphoresis

Potential for Injury: corneal abrasion related to inability to close eye lids secondary to exophthalmus

Potential for Injury related to tremors

Knowledge Deficit: (specify)

examples:

- condition
- treatment regime
- pharmacologic therapy
- eye care
- dietary management
- signs and symptoms of complications

HYPOTHYROIDISM (Myxodoma)

Potential Complications:

Atherosclerotic heart disease *Acute organic psychosis*
Myxedema coma

Alteration in Nutrition: More than Body Requirements related to intake greater than metabolic needs secondary to slowed metabolic rate

Activity Intolerance related to fatigue and weakness secondary to slowed metabolic rate

Alteration in Bowel Elimination: Constipation related to decreased peristaltic action secondary to decreased metabolic rate and decreased physical activity

Impairment of Skin Integrity related to edema and dryness secondary to decreased metabolic rate and infiltration of fluid into interstitial tissues

Alteration in Comfort related to cold intolerance secondary to decreased metabolic rate
Potential Impaired Social Interactions related to listlessness and depression
Impaired Verbal Communication related to slowed speech secondary to enlarged tongue
Knowledge Deficit: (specify)
examples:
condition
treatment regime
dietary management
signs and symptoms of complications
pharmacologic therapy
sensitivity to narcotics, barbiturates, and anesthetic agents

OBESITY

Alteration in Nutrition: More than Body Requirements related to intake greater than metabolic rate (decreased physical activity)
Activity Intolerance related to fatigue and dyspnea related to increased body weight
Ineffective Individual Coping related to increase in food consumption as a response to stressors
Alteration in Health Maintenance related to inadequate exercise program and stress management techniques
Disturbance in Self-Concept related to feelings of self-degradation and the response of others to the condition
Knowledge Deficit: (specify)
examples:
condition
diet therapy
support groups
hazards of overweight condition

PANCREATITIS

Potential Complications:
Shock
Hemorrhagic pancreatitis
Respiratory failure
Pleural effusion
Hypocalcemia
Hyperglycemia
Alteration in Comfort: Pain related to nasogastric suction, distention of pancreatic capsule, and local peritonitis

Potential Fluid Volume Deficit related to decreased intake
secondary to nausea and vomiting
Alteration in Nutrition: Less than Body Requirements
related to vomiting and diet restrictions
Alteration in Bowel Elimination: Diarrhea related to
excessive excretion of fats in stools secondary to
insufficient pancreatic enzymes
Knowledge Deficit (specify)
examples:
disease
contraindications
alcohol
coffee
large meals
dietary management
follow-up care

Gastrointestinal Disorders

Esophageal Disorders
Esophagitis
Hiatal Hernia
Gastroenteritis
Hemorrhoids/Anal Fissure (nonsurgical)
Inflammatory Intestinal Disorders
Diverticulosis
Diverticulitis
Regional Enteritis
Ulcerative Colitis
Peptic Ulcer
Surgical Procedures (see section on Surgical Procedures)
Abdominal Perineal Resection
Colostomy
Ileostomy
Anorectal Surgery
Cholecystectomy
Tonsilectomy
Special Therapies (see section on Diagnostic and
Therapeutic Procedures)
Gastrostomy
Total Parenteral Nutrition

ESOPHAGEAL DISORDERS (Esophagitis, Hiatal hernia)

Potential Complications:
- *Weight loss*
- *Hemorrhage*
- *Gastric ulcers*

Potential Alteration in Nutrition: Less than Body Requirements related to anorexia, heartburn, and dysphagia

Alteration in Comfort related to heartburn, regurgitation, and eructation

Knowledge Deficit: (specify)

examples:
- condition
- dietary management
- hazards of alcohol and tobacco
- positioning after meals
- pharmacologic therapy
- weight reduction (if indicated)

GASTROENTERITIS

Potential Fluid Volume Deficit related to vomiting and diarrhea

Alteration in Comfort related to abdominal cramps, diarrhea, and vomiting

Knowledge Deficit: (specify)

examples:
- condition
- dietary restrictions
- signs and symptoms of complications

HEMORRHOIDS/ANAL FISSURE (Nonsurgical)

Potential Complications:
- *Bleeding*
- *Strangulation*
- *Thrombosis*

Alteration in Comfort related to pain on defecation

Potential Alteration in Bowel Elimination: Constipation related to fear of pain on defecation

Knowledge Deficit: (specify)

examples:
- condition
- bowel routine
- diet instructions
- exercise program
- perianal care

INFLAMMATORY INTESTINAL DISORDERS

(Diverticulosis, Diverticulitis Regional Enteritis, Ulcerative Colitis)

Potential Complications:

Anal fissure
Perianal abscess, fissure, fistula
Anemia
Intestinal obstruction

Alteration in Comfort: Pain related to intestinal inflammatory process
Alteration in Bowel Elimination: Diarrhea related to intestinal inflammatory process
Alteration in Bowel Elimination: Constipation related to inadequate dietary intake of fiber
Potential Impairment of Skin Integrity (perineum): related to diarrhea and chemical irritants
Potential Ineffective Individual Coping: depression related to the chronicity of the condition and the lack of definitive treatment
Alteration in Nutrition: Less than Body Requirements, related to diarrhea, dietary restrictions, and pain with or after eating
Alteration in Health Maintenance: Inadequate stress management, inadequate exercise program
Knowledge Deficit: (specify)
examples:
condition
dietary restrictions
signs and symptoms of complications

PEPTIC ULCER

Potential Complications:

Hemorrhage
Perforation
Pyloric obstruction

Alteration in Comfort: Pain related to lesions secondary to increased gastric secretions
Potential Alteration in Bowel Elimination: Constipation related to diet restrictions and side effects of medications
Possible Ineffective Individual Coping related to excessive uncontrolled internal emotions anger, anxiety, resentment

Knowledge Deficit: (specify)
examples:
condition
dietary restrictions
contraindications
certain medications — tobacco
alcohol — caffeine
signs and symptoms of complications

Renal/Urinary Tract Disorders

Renal Failure
Acute
Chronic (Uremia)
Urinary Tract Infections
Cystitis
Pyelonephritis
Glomerulonephritis
Urolithiasis (Renal Calculi)
Surgical Procedures (see section on Surgical Procedures)
Renal Surgery: General
Percutaneous Nephrostomy
Extracorporeal Renal Surgery
Renal Transplant
Urinary Diversion
Ileal Conduit
Ureterosigmoidostomy
Cutaneous Ureterostomy
Suprapubic Cystostomy
Therapeutic Procedures (see section on Diagnostic and Therapeutic Procedures)
Hemodialysis
Peritoneal Dialysis

RENAL FAILURE (Acute)

Potential Complications:
Fluid overload
Metabolic acidosis
Electrolyte imbalance

Alteration in Nutrition: Less than Body Requirements related to anorexia and dietary restrictions
Potential for Infection related to invasive procedures

Knowledge Deficit: (specify)
  examples:
    disease process
    treatment
    prognosis
    dietary restrictions

RENAL FAILURE (Chronic; Uremia)

See also Peritoneal Dialysis and Hemodialysis if Indicated.

Potential Complications:
  Fluid/electrolyte imbalance
  Hypertension
  Gastrointestinal bleeding
  Hyperparathyroidism
  Pathological fractures
  Malnutrition
  Anemia, thrombocytopenia
  Polyneuropathy (peripheral)
  Decrease in albumin levels
  Congestive heart failure
  Pulmonary edema
  Metabolic acidosis
  Pleural effusion
  Pericarditis

Fluid Volume Excess: peripheral edema related to fluid and electrolyte imbalances secondary to renal dysfunction

Alteration in Nutrition: Less than Body Requirements related to
  examples:
    anorexia
    nausea/vomiting
    loss of taste, smell
    stomatitis
    unpalatable diet

Sexual Dysfunction related to
  examples:
    decreased libido
    impotence
    amenorrhea
    sterility

Disturbance in Self-Concept related to the effects of limitation on achievement of developmental tasks

Potential Social Isolation (individual, family) related to the disability and treatment requirements

Alteration in Comfort related to
  examples:
    fatigue
    headaches
    fluid retention
    anemia

Sexual Dysfunction related to fatigue and decreased libido

Impairment of Skin Integrity related to pruritus, "burning" over lower extremities, and puncture sites (dialysis)

Activity Intolerance related to fatigue secondary to anemia
Impairment of Skin Integrity: pruritus related to the abnormal deposition of calcium secondary to calcium/phosphate imbalance
Knowledge Deficit: (specify)
- examples:
  - condition
  - fluid and sodium restrictions
  - dietary restrictions
    - protein
    - potassium
    - sodium
  - daily recording
    - intake
    - output
    - weights
  - pharmacologic therapy
  - signs/symptoms of complications
  - follow-up visits
  - community resources (support groups)

URINARY TRACT INFECTIONS (Cystitis, Pyelonephritis, Glomerulonephritis)

See also Acute Renal Failure.

Alteration in Comfort: Pain (back, abdominal) related to inflammation and tissue trauma
Alteration in Patterns of Urinary Elimination: dysuria related to inflammation and infection
Potential Alteration in Nutrition: Less than Body Requirements related to anorexia secondary to malaise
Potential Ineffective Individual Coping: depression related to the chronicity of the condition
Knowledge Deficit: (specify)
- examples:
  - prevention of recurrence
    - adequate fluid intake
    - frequent voiding
    - hygiene measures (personal, post-toileting)
    - voiding after sexual activity
  - signs/symptoms of recurrence
  - pharmacologic therapy

UROLITHIASIS (Renal calculi)

Potential Complications:
Pyelonephritis | *Acute renal failure*

Alteration in Comfort related to inflammation secondary to irritation of stone

Alteration in Bowel Elimination: Diarrhea related to renointestinal reflexes

Knowledge Deficit: (specify)
examples:
prevention of recurrence
dietary restrictions
fluid requirements

Neurologic Disorders

- Brain Tumor
- Cerebral Vascular Accident
- Nervous System Disorders (Degenerative, demyelinating, inflammatory)
  - Myasthenia Gravis
  - Multiple Sclerosis
  - Muscular Dystrophy
  - Parkinson's Disease
  - Guillain-Barré Syndrome
  - Amyotrophic Lateral Sclerosis
- Presenile Dementia
  - Altzheimer's Disease
  - Huntington's Disease
- Seizure Disorders (Epilepsy)
- Spinal Cord Injury
- Unconscious Patient
- Surgical Procedures (see section on Surgical Procedures)
  - Cranial Surgery

BRAIN TUMOR

Because this disorder can cause alterations varying from minimal to profound, the following possible nursing diagnoses will reflect individuals with varying degrees of involvement.

See also Surgery (General, Cranial).
See also Cancer.

Potential Complications:
Increased intracranial pressure
Paralysis
Hyperthermia
Motor losses
Sensory losses
Cognitive losses

Potential for Injury related to gait disorders, vertigo and/or visual disturbances, compression/displacement of brain tissue
Sensory Perceptual Alterations: (specify) related to compression/displacement of brain tissue
Anxiety/Fear related to implications of condition and uncertain future
Self Care Deficit: (specify) related to inability/difficulty in performing activities of daily living secondary to sensorimotor impairments
Alteration in Nutrition: Less than Body Requirements related to dysphagia and fatigue
Grieving: denial, anger, depression related to actual/perceived loss of function and uncertain future
Impaired Physical Mobility: upper/lower limbs related to sensorimotor impairment
Alteration in Comfort: headache related to compression/displacement of brain tissue and increased intracranial pressure
Alteration in Family Processes related to the nature of the condition, role disturbances, and uncertain future
Disturbance in Self-Concept related to interruption/failure in achieving developmental tasks (child, adolescence, young adult, middle age)
Potential Fluid Volume Deficit related to vomiting secondary to increased intracranial pressure
Potential for Injury related to impaired/uncontrolled sensorimotor function

CEREBRAL VASCULAR ACCIDENT

Because this disorder can cause alterations varying from minimal to profound, the following possible nursing diagnoses will reflect individuals with varying degrees of involvement.

Potential Complications:
Increased intracranial pressure
Pneumonia
Atelectasis

Sensory Perceptual Alterations: (specify) related to

hypoxia and compression or displacement of brain tissue

Impaired Verbal Communication related to dysarthia and/or aphasia

Potential for Injury related to
examples:
- visual field deficits
- motor deficits
- perception deficits
- inability to perceive environmental hazards

Impaired Physical Mobility related to impaired limb mobility (upper/lower)

Activity Intolerance related to
examples:
- fatigue
- weakness
- inability to tolerate increased activity

Potential Impairment of Skin Integrity related to
examples:
- immobility
- incontinence
- sensory deficits
- motor deficits
- nutritional deficits

Potential Alteration in Nutrition:
Less than Body Requirements, related to dysphagia and self-feeding difficulty

Potential Alteration in Bowel Elimination: Constipation related to prolonged periods of immobility, inadequate fluid intake and inadequate nutritional intake

Potential Alteration in Respiratory Function related to prolonged periods of immobility

Grieving (family, individual) related to the actual or perceived loss of function and inability to meet role responsibilities

Alteration in Patterns of Urinary Elimination:
incontinence related to loss of bladder tone and sphincter control and inability to perceive bladder cues as a result of cerebral dysfunction

Potential Impaired Social Interactions related to difficulty communicating and embarrassment regarding disabilities

Potential Fluid Volume Deficit related to:
examples:
- dysphagia
- difficulty in obtaining fluids
- fatigue
- weakness
- sensorimotor deficits

Potential Impaired Home Maintenance Management

related to altered ability to maintain self at home secondary to sensorimotor/cognitive deficits

Knowledge Deficit: (specify)
examples:
- condition
- pharmacologic therapy
- self-care activities of daily living
- home care
- speech therapy
- exercise program
- community resources
- self-help groups
- signs and symptoms of complications
- skin care
- bowel/bladder program
- reality orientation
- possible behavioral responses
- lability
- regression

NERVOUS SYSTEM DISORDERS (Degenerative, Demyelinating, Inflammatory; Myasthenia Gravis, Multiple Sclerosis, Muscular Dystrophy, Parkinson's Disease, Guillain-Barré Syndrome, Amyotrophic Lateral Sclerosis)

Because the alterations associated with these disorders can range from minimal to profound, the following possible nursing diagnoses will reflect individuals with varying degrees of involvement.

Potential Complications:
- *Renal failure*
- *Pneumonia*
- *Atelectasis*

Disturbance in Self-Concept related to prolonged debilitating condition and interruption in achieving development tasks (adolescence, young adult, middle age)

Impaired Physical Mobility related to muscle dysfunction

Potential for Injury related to
examples:
- visual disturbances
- unsteady gait
- weakness
- uncontrolled movements

Impaired Verbal Communication related to dysarthrias secondary to cranial nerve impairment

Potential Alteration in Nutrition: Less than Body Requirements related to dysphagia/chewing difficulties secondary to cranial nerve impairment

Potential Alteration in Bowel Elimination: Constipation related to immobility

Activity Intolerance related to fatigue and difficulty in performing activities of daily living

Potential Impairment of Skin Integrity related to immobility and sensorimotor deficits

Alteration in Patterns of Urinary Elimination: retention and incontinence related to sensorimotor deficits

Grieving (patient, family) related to the nature of the disease and uncertain prognosis

Sexual Dysfunction (female) related to loss of libido, fatigue and decreased perineal sensation

Sexual Dysfunction (male): impotence related to neurosensory deficits

Potential for Injury related to decreased perception of pain, touch, and temperature

Alteration in Family Processes related to the nature of the disease, role disturbances and uncertain future

Potential Diversional Activity related to inability to perform usual job-related/recreational activities

Potential Social Isolation related to mobility difficulties and associated embarrassment

Home Maintenance Management related to inability/ difficulty in caring for self/home secondary to disability or unavailable or inadequate caretaker

Potential Alteration in Parenting related to impaired ability to perform parenting role secondary to disability

Ineffective Individual Coping: depression related to implications of the disease and its prognosis

Self Care Deficits: (specify) related to

examples:

- headaches
- muscular spasms
- joint pain
- fatigue
- paresis/paralysis

Powerlessness related to inability to control symptoms and the unpredictable nature of the condition (*e.g.*, remissions/exacerbations)

Ineffective Airway Clearance related to impaired ability to cough
Knowledge Deficit:
- examples:
  - condition
  - risks
    - severe fatigue
    - infection
    - cold
    - fever
    - pregnancy
  - exercise program
  - nutritional requirements
  - community services
  - medications
    - schedule
    - side-effects

PRESENILE DEMENTIA (Alzheimer's Disease, Huntington's Disease)

*See also Nervous System Diseases.**

Potential for Injury related to lack of awareness of environmental hazard
Sensory Perceptual Alterations related to an inability to evaluate reality secondary to cerebral neuronal degeneration
Impaired Physical Mobility related to gait instability
Potential Alteration in Family Processes related to effects of condition on relationships, role responsibilities, and finances
Impaired Home Maintenance Management related to inability/difficulty in caring for self/home or inadequate/unavailable caretaker

SEIZURE DISORDERS (Epilepsy)

If the client is a child, see also Development Problems/ Needs

Potential for Injury related to uncontrolled tonic/clonic movements during seizure episode

* Because these disorders can cause alterations similar to the nervous system disorder category, the reader is referred to this section to review additional possible diagnoses.

Potential Social Isolation related to fear of a seizure in public (embarrassment)
Potential Disturbance in Self-Concept related to interruption/failure in achieving developmental tasks (child adolescence, young adult, middle age)
Potential Alteration in Oral Mucous Membrane related to the effects of drug therapy on oral tissue
Fear related to unpredictable nature of seizures and embarrassment
Knowledge Deficit:
- examples:
  - condition
  - medication
    - schedule
    - side effects
  - activity versus rest (balance)
  - care during seizure
  - community resources
  - possible environmental hazards
    - swimming
    - diving
    - operating machinery
  - identification
    - tag
    - card

SPINAL CORD INJURY*

Potential Complications:
- *Accidental extension of injury (acute)*
- *Autonomic dysreflexia (postacute)*
- *Electrolyte imbalance*
- *Spinal shock*
- *Hemorrhage*
- *Respiratory complications*
- *Paralytic ileus*
- *Neurogenic bladder*
- *Hydronephrosis*
- *Gastrointestinal bleeding*
- *Infection (pulmonary, renal)*
- *Thrombophlebitis (deep vein)*
- *Postural hypotension*

Self-Care Deficit: (specify) related to sensorimotor deficits secondary to level of spinal cord injury

* Because disabilities associated with spinal cord injuries can be varied (hemiparesis, quadroparesis, diplegia, monoplegia, triplegia, paraplegia), the nurse will have to clearly specify the individual's limitations in the diagnostic statement.

Impaired Verbal Communication related to impaired ability to speak words secondary to tracheostomy

Fear related to
- examples:
  - abandonment by others
  - changes in role responsibilities
  - effects of injury on life-style
  - multiple tests and procedures
  - separation from support systems

Grieving: denial, anger, depression related to the anticipated losses secondary to sensorimotor deficits

Alteration in Family Processes related to the adjustment requirements for the situation (time, energy, financial, physical care, prognosis)

Potential Impaired Home Maintenance Management related to inadequate resources, housing or impaired caregiver(s)

Potential Social Isolation (individual/family) related to disability or requirements for the caregiver(s)

Potential Alteration in Parenting: abuse, rejection, overprotection related to inadequate resources and coping mechanisms

Disturbance in Self-Concept related to the effects of limitations on achievement of developmental tasks

Potential Fluid Volume Deficit related to difficulty obtaining liquids

Potential Alterations in Nutrition: More than Body Requirements related to imbalance of intake versus activity expenditures

Potential Alterations in Nutrition: Less than Body Requirements related to anorexia and increased metabolic requirements

Potential Diversional Activity Deficit related to the effects of limitations on ability to participate in recreational activities

Potential Alteration in Bowel Elimination: Constipation related to bowel atony, decreased peristalsis, and decreased ability to voluntarily defecate secondary to sensorimotor deficits and immobility

Potential Alteration in Patterns of Urinary Elimination: incontinence, retention related to bladder atony secondary to sensorimotor deficits

Potential Impairment of Skin Integrity related to
examples:
- decreased vascular tone
- immobility
- sensorimotor deficits
- incontinence (bowel, bladder)

Potential for Injury related to impaired ability to control movements and sensorimotor deficits

Potential for Injury: fractures related to bone demineralization secondary to immobility

Potential for Infection related to
examples:
- urinary stasis
- repeated catheterizations
- invasive procedures
  - skeletal tongs
  - tracheostomy
  - venous lines
  - surgical sites

Potential Alteration in Respiratory Function related to
examples:
- immobility
- excessive secretions
- mechanical obstruction

Sexual Dysfunction related to
examples:
- inability to achieve or sustain an erection for intercourse
- limitations on sexual performance
- value conflicts regarding sexual expression
- depression/anxiety
- decreased libido
- altered self-concept
- unwilling/uninformed partner

Knowledge Deficit: (specify)
examples:
- condition
- treatment regime
- rehabilitation
- assistance devices

UNCONSCIOUS INDIVIDUAL

See also Mechanical Ventilation if indicated

Potential Complications:
- *Respiratory insufficiency*
- *Pneumonia*
- *Bladder distention/ incontinence*

Atelectasis
Fluid/electrolyte imbalance
Negative nitrogen balance
Seizures
Stress ulcers
Increased intracranial pressure

Potential for Infection related to immobility and invasive devices (tracheostomy, foley catheter, venous lines)
Potential Impairment of Skin Integrity related to immobility
Potential for Injury: corneal irritation related to corneal drying secondary to open eyes and lower tear production
Anxiety/Fear (family) related to the present state of the individual and the uncertain prognosis
Potential Alteration in Oral Mucous Membrane related to inability to perform mouth care on self and pooling of secretions
Self Care Deficit: total related to unconscious state

Sensory Disorders

- Ophthalmic Disorders
  - Cataracts
  - Detached Retina
  - Glaucoma
  - Inflammations
- Otic Disorders
  - Infections
  - Mastoiditis
  - Trauma
- Surgical Procedures (see section on Surgical Procedures)
  - Ophthalmic Surgery
  - Otic Surgery
    - Stapedectomy
    - Tympanoplasty
    - Myringoplasty
    - Tympanic Mastoidectomy

OPHTHALMIC DISORDERS (Cataracts, Detached Retina, Glaucoma, Inflammations)

See also Ophthalmic Surgery if indicated.

Potential for Injury related to impaired vision secondary to condition or eye patches

Alteration in Comfort: Pain related to
- examples:
  - inflammation
    - lid
    - lacrimal structures
    - conjunctiva
    - uveal tract
    - retina
    - cornea
    - sclera
  - infection
  - increased intraocular pressure
  - ocular tumors

Potential Social Isolation related to fear of injury or embarrassment outside home environment

Potential Impaired Home Maintenance Management related to impaired ability to perform activities of daily living secondary to impaired vision

Self Care Deficit (specify) related to impaired vision

Anxiety/Fear related to the actual or possible loss of vision

Sensory Perceptual Alterations: Visual related to condition or treatment restrictions

Knowledge Deficit: (specify)
- examples:
  - condition
  - eye care
    - patches
    - compresses
  - medications
    - eye drops
    - instillation
  - safety measures
  - activity restrictions
  - follow-up care

OTIC DISORDERS (Infections, Mastoiditis, Trauma)

Potential for Injury related to disturbances of balance and impaired ability to detect environmental hazards

Impaired Verbal Communication related to difficulty understanding others secondary to impaired hearing

Potential Impaired Social Interactions related to difficulty in participating in conversations

Social Isolation related to the lack of contact with others secondary to fear and embarrassment of hearing losses

Alteration in Comfort: Pain related to
- examples:
  - inflammation
  - infection
  - tinnitus
  - vertigo

Sensory Perceptual Alterations: Auditory related to condition or treatment restrictions

Anxiety/Fear related to actual or possible loss of hearing

Knowledge Deficit: (specify)
- examples:
  - condition
  - medications
  - prevention of recurrence
  - hazards
    - swimming
    - air travel
    - showers
  - signs and symptoms of complications
  - hearing aids

Integumentary Disorders

- Dermatologic Disorders
  - Dermatitis
  - Psoriasis
  - Eczema
- Pressure Ulcers
- Skin Infections
  - Impetigo
  - Herpes Zoster
  - Fungal Infections
- Thermal Injuries
  - Burns
  - Severe Hyperthermia

DERMATOLOGIC DISORDERS (Dermatitis, Psoriasis, Eczema)

Impairment of Skin Integrity related to lesions and inflammatory response

Alteration in Comfort: pruritus related to dermal eruptions

Potential Impaired Social Interaction related to fear of embarrassment and negative reactions of others

Potential Disturbance in Self-Concept related to appearance and response of others

Knowledge Deficit: (specify)

examples:

- condition
- topical agents
- contraindications

PRESSURE ULCERS*

Potential for Infection related to susceptibility of open wound

Impairment of Skin Integrity: pressure sores related to

examples:

- skin deficits (edema, obesity, dryness)
- impaired oxygen transport (edema, peripheral anemia)
- chemical/mechanical irritants (casts, radiation, incontinence)
- nutritional deficits
- systemic deficits (infection, cancer, renal or hepatic disorders, diabetes mellitus)
- sensory deficits (confusion, cord injury, neuropathy)
- immobility

Impaired Home Maintenance Management related to complexity of care or unavailable caregiver

* The factors that can contribute to the development of pressure sores are varied and complex; therefore, the nurse must assess for and identify the specific etiologic/contributing factors for the individual.

The following are some situations that contribute to pressure sore development. If the situation is present in the client, the nursing diagnosis can be used.

Alteration in Nutrition: Less than Body Requirements, related to anorexia secondary to (specify)
Impaired Physical Mobility related to (specify)
Fluid Volume Excess: edema related to (specify)
Alteration in Patterns of Urinary Elimination: Incontinence related to (specify)
Sensory Perceptual Alterations: inability to feel or perceive pressure related to (specify)
Knowledge Deficit: (specify)
examples:
causes of pressure ulcers
preventive measures
treatment

SKIN INFECTIONS (Impetigo, Herpes Zoster, Fungal Infections)

Potential Complications (herpes zoster):
Post-herpetic neuralgia
Keratitis
Uveitis
Corneal ulceration
Blindness

Impairment of Skin Integrity related to lesions and pruritus
Alteration in Comfort: pain, pruritus related to dermal eruptions
Potential for Infection to others related to contagious nature of the organism
Knowledge Deficit: (specify)
examples:
condition (causes, course)
prevention
treatments
skin care

THERMAL INJURIES (Burns, Severe Hypothermia)

Acute Period

Potential Complications:
Death
Fluid-loss shock
Fluid overload
Infection/septicemia
Anemia
Negative nitrogen balance
Convulsive disorders

Emboli
Graft rejection
Hypothermia
Hypokalemia/hyperkalemia
Curling's ulcer
Paralytic ileus
Stress diabetes
Adrenal/cortical insufficiency
Pneumonia
Renal failure
Compartmental syndrome
Confusion

Impairment of Skin Integrity related to loss of protective layer secondary to thermal injury
Alteration in Nutrition: Less than Body Requirements related to increased caloric requirement secondary to thermal injury and inability to ingest increased requirements
Alteration in Comfort: Pain related to thermal injury and treatments
Self Care Deficit: (specify) related to impaired range of motion ability secondary to pain and contractures
Fear related to painful procedures and possibility of death
Potential Social Isolation related to infection control measures and separation from family and support systems
Potential Alteration in Bowel Elimination: Constipation related to immobility and effects of pain medication on peristalsis
Sleep Rest Disturbances related to position restrictions, pain, and treatment interruptions
Potential Sensory Perceptual Alterations related to examples:
excessive environmental stimuli
stress
imposed immobility
sleep deprivation
protective isolation
Grieving (family, individual) related to actual or perceived impact of injury on life (appearance, relationships, occupation)
Potential Impairment of Skin Integrity: pressure ulcer related to immobility

Postacute Period

If individual is a child, see also Developmental Problems/Needs.

Potential Complications: same as acute
contractures

Diversional Activity Deficit related to monotony of confinement
Potential Social Isolation related to embarrassment and the response of others to injury
Powerlessness related to inability to control present situation
Disturbances in Self-Concept related to the effects of the thermal injury on achieving developmental tasks (child, adolescent, adult)
Potential Impaired Physical Mobility: contractures related to loss of motion, scarring or reluctance to move secondary to pain
Fear related to uncertain future and effects of injury on life style, relationships, occupation
Impaired Home Maintenance Management related to long-term requirements of treatments
Knowledge Deficit: (specify)
- examples:
  - Condition
  - Treatment
    - surgery
    - whirlpool
  - Nutritional requirements
  - Pain management
  - Home care
  - Rehabilitation
  - Community services

Musculoskeletal/Connective Tissue Disorders

- Fractured Jaw
- Fractures
- Low back pain
- Osteomyelitis
- Osteoporosis
- Rheumatic Diseases
- Surgical Procedures (See section on Surgical Procedures)
  - Amputation

Arthroplasty (Hip, Knee, Ankle)
Arthroscopy, Arthrotomy, Menisectomy, Bunionectomy
Fracture Hip
Laminectomy
Therapeutic Procedures (See section on Diagnostic and Therapeutic Procedures)
Casts

FRACTURED JAW

Potential Complications:
aspiration
infection
Alteration in Oral Mucous Membrane related to difficulty in performing oral hygiene secondary to fixation devices
Impaired Verbal Communication related to fixation devices
Alteration in Comfort: Pain related to tissue trauma
Potential Alteration in Nutrition: Less than Body Requirements related to inability to ingest solid food secondary to fixation devices
Knowledge Deficit: (specify)
examples:
mouth care
nutritional requirements
signs and symptoms of infection
procedure for emergency wire cutting (*e.g.*, vomiting)

FRACTURES

See also Casts.
Potential Complications:
Neurovascular (paresis, paralysis)
Fat embolism syndrome
Shock (hemorrhagic, hypovolemic)
Misalignment
Osteomyelitis
Compartmental syndrome
Contracture
Alteration in Comfort: Pain related to tissue trauma
Potential Impairment of Skin Integrity related to

mechanical irritants/compression secondary to casts and traction

Impairment of Skin Integrity related to invasive fixation devices

Self Care Deficits: (specify) related to impaired ability to use upper/lower limb secondary to immobilization device

Potential for Injury related to incorrect use of ambulation assistance devices (walker, crutches)

Diversional Activity Deficit related to boredom of confinement secondary to immobilization devices

Potential for Infection: urinary tract related to immobility secondary to fixation devices

Potential Impaired Home Maintenance Management related to:

examples:

- fixation device
- impaired physical mobility
- unavailable support system

Alteration in Family Processes related to the difficulty of ill person to assume role responsibilities secondary to limited motion

Impaired Physical Mobility related to fixation devices

Potential Alteration in Bowel Elimination: Constipation related to decreased physical activity

Potential Alteration in Respiratory Function related to immobility secondary to traction or other fixation devices

Knowledge Deficit: (specify)

examples:

- condition
- cast care
- use of assistance devices
  - cane
  - crutches
  - walker
- signs and symptoms of complications
  - numbness
  - pallor
  - decreased sensation
- limitations

LOW BACK PAIN

Potential Complications:
Herniated nucleus pulposus

Alteration in Comfort: Pain related to:
examples:
acute lumbosacral strain
unstable lumbosacral ligaments
weak muscles
osteoarthritis of spine
spinal stenosis
intervertebral disk program

Impaired Physical Mobility related to decreased mobility and flexibility secondary to muscle spasm

Potential Ineffective Individual Coping: depression related to the effects of chronic pain on life-style

Potential Alteration in Family Processes related to the impaired ability of individual to meet role responsibilities (financial, home, social)

Knowledge Deficit: (specify)
examples:
condition
exercise program
noninvasive pain relief methods
relaxation
imagery
proper posture and body mechanics

OSTEOMYELITIS

Potential Complications:
Bone abscess

Alteration in Comfort: Pain related to soft tissue edema secondary to infection

Impaired Physical Mobility related to limited range of motion of affected bone

Knowledge Deficit: (specify)
examples:
condition
etiology
course
pharmacologic therapy
nutritional requirements
pain management
signs and symptoms of complications

OSTEOPOROSIS

Potential Complications:
- *Fractures*
- *Kyphosis*
- *Paralytic ileus*

Alteration in Comfort: Pain related to muscle spasm and fractures
Alteration in Health Maintenance related to insufficient daily physical activity
Alteration in Nutrition: Less than Body Requirements, related to inadequate dietary intake of calcium, protein, and vitamin D
Impaired Physical Mobility related to limited range of motion secondary to skeletal changes
Fear related to unpredictable nature of condition
Potential for Injury: fractures related to porous bones secondary to disease process
Knowledge Deficit: (specify)
- examples:
  - condition
    - etiology
    - course
  - nutritional therapy
  - activity program
  - safety precautions
  - prevention

RHEUMATIC DISEASES

Alteration in Comfort: Pain related to inflammatory response and joint immobility (stiffness)
Activity Intolerance related to fatigue and stiffness
Self Care Deficits: (specify) related to loss of motion, muscle weakness, pain, stiffness, or fatigue
Ineffective Individual Coping related to the stress imposed by exacerbations (unpredictable)
Alteration in Health Maintenance: stress management
Disturbances in Self-Concept related to physical and psychological changes imposed by the disease
Impaired Home Maintenance Management related to impaired ability to perform household responsibilities secondary to limited mobility
Sleep Pattern Disturbance related to pain

Impaired Home Maintenance Management related to fatigue and impaired mobility
Impaired Physical Mobility related to pain and limited motion of limbs
Sexual Dysfunction related to difficulty assuming position (female), fatigue, or pain
Potential Social Isolation related to ambulation difficulty and fatigue
Alteration in Family Processes related to difficulty/inability of ill person to assume role responsibilities secondary to fatigue and limited motion
Knowledge Deficit: (specify)
examples:
- condition
- rest versus exercise
- self-help groups
- assistance devices
- quackery
- heat therapy
- pharmacologic therapy

Infectious/Immunodeficient Disorders

Lupus Erythematosus (Systemic)
Meningitis/Encephalitis
Sexually Transmitted Infectious Diseases
- Venereal Disease
- Herpes
- Acquired Immune Deficiency Syndrome (AIDS)

LUPUS ERYTHEMATOSUS (Systemic)

See also Rheumatic Diseases.
See also Corticosteroid Therapy.
Potential Complications:
- *Renal failure of corticosteroid therapy*
- *Pericarditis*
- *Pleuritis*

Powerlessness related to the unpredictable course (remissions, exacerbations)
Ineffective Individual Coping: depression related to unpredictable course and altered appearance

Potential Social Isolation related to embarrassment and the response of others to appearance
Potential Disturbance in Self-Concept related to inability to achieve developmental tasks secondary to the disabling condition
Knowledge Deficit: (specify)
examples:
condition
rest/activity balance
pharmacologic therapy

MENINGITIS/ENCEPHALITIS

Potential Complications:
Fluid/electrolyte imbalance
Cerebral edema
Adrenal damage
Circulatory collapse
Hemorrhage
Convulsions
Septicemia
Alkalosis
Increased intracranial pressure

Potential for Infection to others related to contagious nature of organism
Alteration in Comfort: headache, fever, neck pain related to meningeal irritation
Activity Intolerance related to fatigue and malaise secondary to infection
Potential Impairment of Skin Integrity related to immobility, dehydration, and diaphoresis
Potential Alteration in Oral Mucous Membrane related to dehydration and impaired ability to perform mouth care
Potential Alteration in Nutrition: Less than Body Requirements related to anorexia, fatigue, nausea, and vomiting
Potential Alteration in Respiratory Function related to immobility and pain
Potential for Injury related to restlessness and disorientation secondary to meningeal irritation
Alteration in Family Processes related to critical nature of the situation and uncertain prognosis
Anxiety/Fear related to treatments, environment, and risk of death
Knowledge Deficit: (specify)
examples:
condition
treatments
signs and symptoms of complications

pharmacologic therapy
rest/activity balance
follow-up care
prevention of recurrence

SEXUALLY TRANSMITTED INFECTIOUS DISEASES (Venereal Diseases, Herpes, Acquired Immune Deficiency Syndrome [AIDS])

Potential for Infection to Others related to the contagious agents
Fear related to nature of the condition and its implications on life style
Grieving: anger, depression related to the chronicity of the condition (herpes) or the poor prognosis (AIDS)
Alteration in Comfort related to the inflammatory process
Powerlessness related to incurable nature of the condition
Social Isolation related to fear of transmitting the disease to others
Knowledge Deficit: (specify)
examples:
condition
modes of transmission
consequences of repeated infections
prevention of recurrences

Neoplastic Disorders

Cancer (General, Applies to malignancies in varied sites and stages)
Colon-Rectal Cancer (Additional Diagnoses)
See also Surgical Procedures and Diagnostic and Therapeutic Procedures
Mastectomy
Radical Neck Dissection
Pelvic Exenteration
Chemotherapy
Radiation Therapy
Abdominoperineal Resection

CANCER (General)

Alteration in Oral Mucous Membranes related to
examples:
- disease process
- therapy
  - radiation
  - chemotherapy
- inadequate oral hygiene
- altered nutritional/hydration status

Potential Sexual Dysfunction related to
examples:
- fear
- grieving
- changes in body image
- anatomic changes
- pain, fatigue (treatments, disease)
- change in role responsibilities

Alteration in Comfort related to disease process and treatments

Alteration in Bowel Elimination: Diarrhea related to
examples:
- disease process
- chemotherapy
- radiation
- medications

Alteration in Bowel Elimination: Constipation related to
examples:
- disease process
- chemotherapy
- radiation therapy
- immobility
- dietary intake
- medications

Disturbance in Self-Concept related to
examples:
- anatomic changes
- role disturbances
- uncertain future
- disruption of life-style

Self Care Deficits: (specify) related to fatigue, pain, or depression

Potential for Infection related to altered immune system

Alteration in Nutrition: Less than Body Requirements related to anorexia, fatigue, nausea, and vomiting, secondary to disease process and treatments

Potential for Injury: physical falls related to
examples:
- disorientation

weakness
sensory/perceptual deterioration
skeletal/muscle deterioration

Potential Impairment of Skin Integrity related to
examples:
immobility
altered nutrition status
altered circulation
altered sensation
excretions/secretions
radiation therapy

Alteration in Patterns of Urinary Elimination: incontinence related to disease process

Potential Fluid Volume Deficit related to
examples:
altered ability/desire to obtain fluids
weakness
vomiting
diarrhea
depression
fatigue

Potential Impaired Home Maintenance Management related to
examples:
lack of knowledge
lack of resources
support system
equipment
financial
motor deficits
sensory deficits
cognitive deficits
emotional deficits

Potential Impaired Social Interactions related to the fear of rejection or actual rejection of others after diagnosis

Potential for Injury related to bleeding tendencies and thrombocytopenia

Potential Alteration in Respiratory Function related to fatigue, pain, and immobility

Powerlessness related to inability to control situation

Alteration in Family Process related to
examples:
stress of diagnosis/treatments
role disturbances
uncertain future

Grieving (family, individual): anger, denial, depression related to actual, perceived, or anticipated losses associated with the diagnosis

Knowledge Deficit: (specify)
- examples:
  - disease
  - misconceptions
  - treatments
  - home care
  - support agencies
    - self-help groups
    - American Cancer Society
    - hospital associations

COLON/RECTAL CANCER

(Additional Diagnoses)

See also Cancer (General).

Impairment of Skin Integrity related to stoma and its effects on adjacent skin surfaces

Potential Sexual Dysfunction (male) related to inability to have or sustain an erection secondary to surgical procedure on perineal structures

Knowledge Deficit: (specify)
- examples:
  - preoperative procedures
  - postoperative procedures
  - ostomy care
    - Appliances
    - Irrigations
  - dietary management
  - signs and symptoms of complications

Surgical Procedures

General Surgery

Abdominoperineal Resection

- Colostomy
- Ileostomy

Amputation
Aneurysm Resection, Abdominal Aortic
Anorectal Surgery
Arterial Occlusion with Graft of Lower Extremity

- Femoral
- Popliteal
- Aortic
- Iliac

Arthroplasty (Total Hip, Knee, or Ankle Replacement)
Arthroscopy, Arthrotomy, Menisectomy, Bunionectomy
Carotid Endarterectomy
Cesarean Section
Cholecystectomy
Cranial Surgery
Dilatation and Curettage (D&C)
Fractured Hip
Hysterectomy (Vaginal, Abdominal)
Laminectomy
Mastectomy
Myocardial Revascularization (Coronary Artery Bypass)
Ophthalmic Surgery
Otic Surgery

- Stapedectomy
- Tympanoplasty
- Myringotomy
- Tympanic Mastoidectomy

Pelvic Exenteration
Radical Neck Dissection (Laryngectomy)
Renal Surgery (General)

- Percutaneous Nephrostomy/Extracorporeal Renal Surgery

Renal Transplant
Thoracic Surgery
Tonsillectomy
Transurethral Resection

- Prostate (Benign Hypertrophy or Cancer)
- Bladder Tumor

Urinary Diversion

- Ilial Conduit
- Ureterosigmoidostomy
- Cutaneous Ureterostomy
- Suprapubic Cystostomy

GENERAL SURGERY

Preoperative Period

Anxiety related to surgical experience and the unpredictable outcome

Knowledge Deficit: (specify)

- examples:
  - preoperative procedures
    - surgical permit
    - diagnostic studies
    - foley catheter
    - diet and fluid restrictions
    - medications
    - skin preparation
    - waiting area for family
  - postoperative procedure
    - disposition (recovery room, intensive care unit)
    - medications for pain
    - coughing-turning-leg exercises
    - tubes/drain placement
    - NPO/diet restrictions
    - bedrest

Postoperative Period

Potential Complications:

- *Urinary retention*
- *Hemorrhage*
- *Hypovolemia/shock*
- *Renal failure*
- *Pneumonia (stasis)*
- *Infection*
- *Thrombophlebitis*
- *Paralytic ileus*
- *Evisceration*
- *Dehiscence*

Potential for Infection: wound related to the destruction of the first line of defense against bacterial invasion

Potential Alteration in Respiratory Function related to postanesthesia state, postoperative immobility, and pain

Alteration in Comfort: Pain related to surgical intervention

Activity Intolerance related to pain and fatigue

Self-Care Deficits: (specify) related to limited mobility and pain

Potential Alteration in Bowel Elimination: Constipation related to decreased peristalsis secondary to the effects of anesthesia, immobility, and pain medication

Alteration in Nutrition: Less than Body Requirements related to increased protein/vitamin requirements for wound healing and decreased intake secondary to pain, nausea, vomiting, and diet restrictions

Knowledge Deficit: (specify)
examples:
- home care
- incisional care
- signs and symptoms of complications
- activity restriction
- follow-up care

ABDOMINOPERINEAL RESECTION

(Colostomy, Ileostomy)

See also Cancer (General)
See also Surgery (General).

Preoperative Surgery

Knowledge Deficit: (specify)
examples:
- stoma (appearance, care, site)
- postoperative care

Postoperative Period

Potential for Infection: wound related to fecal contamination

Potential Impairment of Skin Integrity: stoma related to erythema secondary to improper location, improper appliance, or sensitivity to appliance material

Disturbance in Self-Concept related to effects of ostomy on self and relationship with others

Possible Sexual Dysfunction (male) related to impotence secondary to surgical disruption of perineal structures

Potential Sexual Dysfunction related to altered self-concept and change in appearance

Potential Social Isolation related to fear of loss of colostomy control, accident, or odor

Grieving (client, family) related to the implications of cancer and change in body functions

Knowledge Deficit: (specify)
examples:
- condition
- perineal wound care

skin care
irritations
odor control
signs and symptoms of complications
community resources (United Ostomy Association)

AMPUTATION

See Surgery (General).

Postoperative Period

Potential Complications:
Edema
Hemorrhage
Infection
Contractures/muscle atrophy

Grieving related to loss of limb and its effects on life-style
Impaired Home Maintenance Management related to architectural barriers
Alteration in Comfort: Pain related to surgical amputation and phantom pain
Potential Disturbance in Self-Concept related to loss of body part
Fear related to surgical procedure, change in life-style, and resultant disability
Potential Alteration in Family Process related to change in life-style (role responsibilities, financial, occupational)
Impaired Physical Mobility related to altered gait
Potential for Injury related to altered gait or improper use or fit of assistance devices
Knowledge Deficit: (specify)
examples:
wound care
exercises
gait training
prosthesis
Use
Maintenance

ANEURYSM RESECTION (Abdominal Aortic)

See Surgery (General).

Postoperative Period

Potential Complications:
- *Cardiocirculatory (hypo- /hypertension, increased cardiac workload, arrhythmias, electrolyte imbalance, thrombus/embolus formation, hemorrhage, compartmental syndrome, thrombophlebitis)*
- *Graft (constriction, occlusion, disruption of anastomosis, arterial spasm)*
- *Renal insufficiency*
- *Paralytic ileus*
- *Anticoagulant therapy*

Alteration in Family Processes related to disruption of family life, fear of outcome (death, disability), and stressful environment (intensive care unit)

Knowledge Deficit: (specify)
examples:
- home care
- follow-up care
- wound care
- anticoagulant therapy

ANORECTAL SURGERY

See also Surgery (General).

Preoperative Period (see Hemorroids or Anal Fissure)

Postoperative Period

Potential Complications:
- *Hemorrhage*
- *Urinary retention*

Alteration in Comfort: Pain related to surgical incision and spasms (sphincter, muscle)

Potential Alteration in Bowel Elimination: Constipation related to failure to respond to cues for defecation for fear of pain

Potential for Infection: anal area related to surgical incision and fecal contamination

Knowledge Deficit: (specify)
examples:
- wound care
- prevention of recurrence

nutritional requirements
  diet
  fluid
exercise program
signs and symptoms of complications

ARTERIAL OCCLUSION WITH GRAFT OF LOWER EXTREMITY

(Femoral, Popliteal, Aortic, Iliac)

See also Surgery (General).
See also Anticoagulant Therapy

Postoperative Period

Potential Complications:
- *Constriction of site*
- *Occlusion*
- *Disruption of anastomosis*
- *Hemorrhage*

Knowledge Deficit: (specify)
  examples:
    risk factors
    foot care
    incision care
    signs of complications
    follow-up care
    implications of anticoagulant therapy
    medications
    activity restrictions

ARTHROPLASTY (Total Hip, Knee, or Ankle Replacement)

Preoperative Period

See also Surgery (General).
  Knowledge Deficit: use of trapeze

Postoperative Period

Potential Complications:
- *Fat emboli*
- *Hematoma formation*
- *Infection*
- *Dislocation of joint*
- *Stress fractures*
- *Neurovascular alterations*
- *Synovial herniation*
- *Thromboemboli formation*

Potential Impairment of Skin Integrity related to immobility and incision
Activity Intolerance related to fatigue, pain, and impaired gait
Impaired Home Maintenance Management related to postoperative flexion restrictions
Potential Alteration in Bowel Elimination: Constipation related to activity restriction
Potential for Injury related to altered gait assistance devices
Knowledge Deficit: (specify)
- examples:
  - activity restrictions
  - use of supportive devices
    - walker
    - crutches
    - canes
  - rehabilitative program
  - follow-up care
  - apparel restrictions
  - signs of complications
  - follow-up care
  - supportive services
  - prevention of infection

ARTHROSCOPY, ARTHROTOMY, MENISCECTOMY, BUNIONECTOMY

See also Surgery (General).

Preoperative Period

Knowledge Deficit: crutch walking and leg exercises

Postoperative Period

Potential Complications:
- *Hematoma formation*
- *Neurovascular impairments*
- *Hemorrhage*
- *Effusion*

Knowledge Deficit: (specify)
- examples:
  - home care
  - incision care
  - activity restrictions

signs of complications
follow-up care

CAROTID ENDARTERECTOMY

See also Surgery (General).

Postoperative Period

Potential Complications:
Circulatory (cerebral vascular accident, hemorrhage, hypo- /hypervolemia, thrombus/embolus formation)
Tracheal deviation
Laryngeal edema
Facial nerve impairment
Seizures

Potential for Injury related to syncope
Knowledge Deficit: (specify)
examples:
risk factors
smoking
diet
obesity
activity restrictions
surgical site care
signs of complications
follow-up care

CESAREAN SECTION

See General Surgery.
See Postpartum Period.

CHOLECYSTECTOMY

See also Surgery (General).

Preoperative Period

Potential Complications:
Peritonitis
Nonfunctioning nasogastric tube

Potential Alteration in Respiratory Function related to high abdominal incision and splinting secondary to pain

Potential Alteration in Oral Mucous Membrane related to NPO state and mouth breathing secondary to nasogastric tube

CRANIAL SURGERY

See also Surgery (General).
See also Brain Tumor for pre- /postoperative care.
Potential Complications:
- *Increased intracranial pressure*
- *Seizures*
- *Respiratory insufficiency*
- *Hypo- /hypertension*
- *Fluid/electrolyte imbalances*
- *Cranial nerve dysfunction (infratentorial)*
- *Cardiac arrhythmias (infratentorial)*
- *Gastrointestinal bleeding*
- *Meningitis/encephalitis*

DILATATION AND CURETTAGE (D&C)

See also Surgery (General; pre- and post-).

Postoperative Period

Potential Complications:
- *Hemorrhage*

Knowledge Deficit: (specify)
examples:
- condition
- home care
- signs and symptoms of complications
- activity restrictions

FRACTURED HIP

See also Surgery (General).

Preoperative Period

Potential Complication:
- *Improper alignment of immobilization devices*

Alteration in Comfort: pain related to trauma and muscle spasms
Knowledge Deficit: use of trapeze

Postoperative Period

Potential Complications:
- *Dislocation of hip joint*
- *Avascular necrosis of femoral head*

Self-Care Deficit: (specify) related to activity restrictions
Knowledge Deficit: (specify)
- examples:
  - exercises
  - activity restrictions
  - home care
  - surgical site care
  - follow-up care
  - supportive services
  - ambulation assistance devices
    - crutches
    - walker

HYSTERECTOMY (Vaginal, Abdominal)

See also Surgery (General).

Postoperative Period

Potential Complications:
- *Vaginal bleeding (postpacking removal)*
- *Urinary retention (postcatheter removal)*
- *Fistula formation*
- *Deep vein thrombosis*
- *Trauma (ureter, bladder, rectal)*

Potential for Infection related to surgical intervention and urinary catheter
Potential Disturbance in Self-Concept related to implications of the loss of body part
Potential Sexual Dysfunction related to the personal significance of the loss of body part and the implications of loss on life-style
Grieving: depression related to loss of body part and child-bearing ability
Knowledge Deficit: (specify)
- examples:
  - perineal/incisional care
  - signs of complications
  - activity restrictions
    - sexual
    - activities of daily living
    - occupational
  - loss of menses
  - follow-up care (routine gynecological exams)

LAMINECTOMY

See also Surgery (General).

Preoperative Period

Anxiety/Fear related to the possibility of postoperative paralysis
Knowledge Deficit: (specify)
examples:
postoperative care
positioning
monitoring
logrolling

Postoperative Period

Potential Complications:
Neurosensory impairments
Bowel/bladder dysfunction
Cord edema
Skeletal malalignment
Cerebral spinal fluid leakage
Hematoma

Potential for Injury related to postural hypotension
Alteration in Comfort: Pain related to muscle spasms (back, thigh) secondary to irritation of nerves during surgery
Impaired Physical Mobility related to treatment restrictions
Potential Diversional Activity Deficit related to monotony of immobility
Self-Care Deficit: (specify) related to activity restrictions
Knowledge Deficit: (specify)
examples:
activity restrictions
immobilization device
exercises

MASTECTOMY

See also Cancer (General).
See also Surgery (General).

Preoperative Period

Fear related to diagnosis of cancer and future implications

Postoperative Period

Potential Complications:

Edema formation

Neurovascular deficits

Potential Fluid Volume Excess related to lymphedema secondary to surgical intervention

Self-Care Deficit (specify) related to impaired mobility of upper limb and limited range of motion

Potential for Injury related to vascular, lymphatic alteration of upper limb

Disturbance in Self-Concept related to loss of body part (breast) and lymphedema

Potential Sexual Dysfunction related to loss of body part and fear of response of partner

Potential Social Isolation related to edema formation and fear of response of others

Knowledge Deficit: (specify)

- examples:
  - condition
  - home care
    - arm exercises
    - wound care
  - self-breast exam
  - hazards to affected arm
    - injections
    - pressure
  - community services
    - Reach for Recovery
    - apparel

MYOCARDIAL REVASCULARIZATION

(Coronary Artery Bypass)

See also Surgery (General).
See also Mechanical Ventilation.
See also Thoracic Surgery.

Postoperative Period

Potential Complications:

Death

Arrhythmias (ventricular, rate, junctional, rhythm)

Low cardiac output syndrome

Cardiac tamponade

Respiratory failure

Hypertension/ hypotension
Hemorrhage
Vasodilatation
Myocardial infarction (perioperative)
Pulmonary embolism
Renal failure
Cerebrovascular accident (embolis/thrombus)
Hypovolemia

Alteration in Comfort: Pain related to surgical incisions, drainage tube, and invasive catheters
Anxiety/Fear related to intensive environment of critical care unit and potential for complications
Impaired Verbal Communication related to endotracheal tube (temporary)
Sleep/Rest Disturbance related to interruptions (noise, treatments, activity)
Alteration in Self-Concept related to the symbolic meaning of the heart
Alteration in Family Processes related to disruption of family life, fear of outcome (death, disability) and stressful environment (ICU)
Knowledge Deficit: (specify)
examples:
- condition
- pain management
  - angina
  - incisional
- incisional care
- risk factors
  - smoking
  - diet
  - obesity
- restrictions
  - activity
  - sexual
- stress management techniques
- signs and symptoms of complications
- follow-up care
- pharmacologic care
- nutritional therapy
- exercise program

OPHTHALMIC SURGERY

See also Surgery (General).

Preoperative Periods

Knowledge Deficit:
examples:
postoperative positioning
postoperative eye care/bandaging
postoperative activity restrictions
positioning
bending
stooping
straining
intraoperative procedure

Fear/Anxiety related to having surgery with a local anesthetic, possible loss of vision, and fear of pain during procedure

Potential Sensory Perceptual Alterations related to impaired vision

Potential for Injury related to impaired vision and unfamiliar environment

Postoperative Periods

Potential Complications:

Swelling | *Increased pain*
Eye damage | *Change in vision*

Sensory Perceptual Alterations related to impaired vision secondary to bandages or lack of availability of visual aides, such as cataract glasses

Potential for Injury related to impaired vision and unfamiliar environment

Disturbance in Self-Concept related to altered appearance secondary to surgery

Diversional Activity Deficits related to inability to participate in recreational activities secondary to impaired vision

Knowledge Deficit: (specify)
examples:
activity restriction
coughing
eye movements
stooping
straining
bending
swimming
lifting heavy objects

eye care
signs and symptoms of complications
pharmacologic therapy

OTIC SURGERY (Stapedectomy, Tympanoplasty, Myringotomy, Tympanic Mastoidectomy)

See also General Surgical Plan.

Preoperative Period

Anxiety/Fear related to the possibility of greater loss of hearing after surgery

Postoperative Period

Potential Complications:

Hemorrhage
Facial paralysis
Infection
Impaired hearing/deafness

Sensory Perceptual Alteration: Auditory related to condition and postoperative bandages
Impaired Verbal Communication related to decreased hearing
Potential Social Isolation related to the embarrassment of not being able to hear when in a social setting
Potential for Injury related to vertigo condition
Knowledge Deficit: (specify)
examples:
- signs and symptoms of complications
  - facial nerve injury
  - vertigo
  - tinnitus
  - gait disturbances
  - ear discharge
- ear care
- contradictions, postoperative period
  - swimming
  - shampooing
  - air flights
  - showering
  - nose blowing
  - sneezing
  - coughing
  - straining
- follow-up care

PELVIC EXENTERATION

See also Cancer (General).
See also Surgery (General).
See also Abdominal–Perineal Resection (Total).

Preoperative Period

Knowledge Deficit:
procedure
postoperative care

Postoperative Period

Potential Complications:
Infection
Paralytic ileus
Urinary stasis

Alteration in Comfort: Pain related to surgical intervention and metastasis
Grieving: denial, anger, depression related to loss of body parts and function and effects on life-style and relationships
Fear related to the possibility of reoccurrence of cancer
Potential Sexual Dysfunction related to
examples:
Altered sexual function
Feelings of being undesirable
Partner's negative response (actual or perceived)
Physiological limitations
Potential Impaired Home Maintenance Management related to effects of debilitating disease and surgery on ability to maintain home
Self-Care Deficit: (specify) related to pain, fatigue, and decreased motivation secondary to depression
Alteration in Family Processes related to the effects of hospitalization, disease process, surgical intervention and fears of reoccurrence on relationships and ability to meet role responsibilities
Knowledge Deficit: (specify)
examples:
signs and symptoms of complications
pharmacologic therapy
home care
community services

RADIAL NECK DISSECTION (laryngectomy)

Preoperative Period

See also Surgery (General).
See also Cancer (General).

Anxiety related to impending surgery and implications of condition on life-style
Knowledge Deficit: (specify)
examples:
postoperative disposition (intensive care unit)
ability to communicate
reading
writing skills
tracheostomy

Postoperative Period

Potential Complications:

Hypoxia	*Tracheal edema*
Carotid rupture	*Cranial nerve injury*
Hemorrhage	*Infection*

Ineffective Airway Clearance related to increased secretions secondary to tracheostomy
Potential Alteration in Nutrition: Less than Body Requirements related to dysphagia secondary to surgical intervention
Potential for Infection: tracheostomy site, related to excessive pooling of secretions and bypassing of upper respiratory defenses
Potential Impaired Physical Mobility: shoulder and neck motion, related to muscle trauma secondary to surgery
Alteration in Oral Mucous Membrane related to excessive secretions or xerostomia
Impaired Verbal Communications related to inability to speak secondary to tracheostomy
Alteration in Self-Concept related to disfiguring surgery and response of others to disfigurement
Potential Sexual Dysfunction related to change in appearance and responses of others to condition
Sensory Perceptual Alterations: Olfactory, related to neural sensory deficits secondary to surgery

Grieving: anger, depression related to loss of voice, olfactory sense and previous appearance
Potential for Injury: aspiration related to tracheostomy
Knowledge Deficit: (specify)
- examples:
  - condition
  - home care
    - oral hygiene
    - suctioning techniques
    - tracheostomy care
    - humidification
  - contraindications (lifting)
  - signs and symptoms of complications
    - swelling
    - pain
    - difficulty swallowing
    - purulent sputum
  - follow-up care
  - identificiation card/tag
  - esophageal breathing
  - community services (American Cancer Society)

RENAL SURGERY (General; Percutaneous Nephrostomy, Extracorporeal Renal Surgery, Nephrectomy)

See also Surgery (General).
Potential Complications:
- *Hemorrhage*
- *Shock*
- *Paralytic ileus*
- *Pneumothorax*
- *Of nephrostomy tube (calculi, fistulae, kinks)*

Alteration in Comfort: Pain related to distention of renal capsule and incision
Potential Alteration of Respiratory Function related to pain on breathing and coughing secondary to location of incision
Knowledge Deficit: (specify)
- examples:
  - nephrostomy care
  - signs and symptoms of complications

RENAL TRANSPLANT

See also Corticosteroid Therapy
See also Surgery (General)
Potential Complications:
- *Hemodynamic instability*
- *Hypervolemia/hypovolemia*
- *Hypertension/hypotension*
- *Renal failure (donor kidney)*
  - *examples:*
    - *ischemic damage prior to implantation*
    - *hematoma*
    - *rupture of anastomosis*
    - *bleeding at anastomosis*
    - *renal vein thrombosis*
    - *renal artery stenosis*
    - *blockage of ureter (kinks, clots)*
    - *kinking of ureter, renal artery*
- *Rejection of donor tissue*
- *Excessive Immunosuppression*
- *Electrolyte imbalances (potassium, phosphate)*
- *Deep vein thrombosis*

Potential for Infection related to altered immune system secondary to medications

Potential Alteration in Oral Mucous Membrane related to increased susceptibility to infection secondary to immunosuppression

Potential Disturbance in Self-Concept related to transplant experience and potential for rejection

Fear related to possibility of rejection and dying

Potential Noncompliance related to the complexity of treatment regime (diet, medications, record keeping, weight, blood pressure, urine testing) and euphoria (post-transplant)

Knowledge Deficit: (specify)
- examples:
  - prevention of infection
    - personal hygiene
    - wound care
    - avoidance of contagious agents
  - activity progression
  - dietary management
  - daily recording

intake
output
weights
urine testing
blood pressure
temperature
pharmacologic therapy
purpose
timing
dosage
precautionary measures
potential adverse effects
daily urine testing (protein)
signs/symptoms of rejection/infection
avoidance of pregnancy
follow-up care
community resources

THORACIC SURGERY

See also Surgery (General)
See also Mechanical Ventilation

Preoperative Period

Anxiety/Fear related to possible respiratory difficulty postsurgery
Knowledge Deficit: (specify)
examples:
drainage devices
mechanical ventilation

Postoperative Period

Potential Complications:
Atelectasis
Pneumonia
Respiratory insufficiency
Complications of chest drainage
Pneumothorax
Hemorrhage
Pulmonary embolus
Subcutaneous emphysema
Mediastinal shift

Ineffective Airway Clearance related to difficulty in coughing secondary to pain
Alteration in Comfort: Pain related to surgical intervention and drainage tube(s)
Activity Intolerance related to reduction in exercise capacity secondary to loss of alveolar ventilation

Impaired Physical Mobility: arm/shoulder related to muscle trauma secondary to surgery and position restrictions
Knowledge Deficit: (specify)
examples:
- condition
- pain management
- shoulder/arm exercises
- incisional care
- breathing exercises
- splinting
- environmental hazards
  - dust
  - smoke
  - irritating chemicals
  - crowds during upper respiratory epidemics
- prevention of infection
- nutritional needs
- rest versus activity
- respiratory toilet
- follow-up care

TONSILLECTOMY

See also Surgery (General).
Potential Complications:
Airway obstruction *Aspiration*
Hemorrhage
Potential Fluid Volume Deficit related to decreased fluid intake secondary to pain on swallowing
Potential Alteration in Nutrition: Less than Body Requirements related to decreased intake secondary to pain on swallowing
Knowledge Deficit: (specify)
examples:
- rest requirements
- nutritional needs
  - soft foods
  - fluids
- signs and symptoms of complications (hemorrhage)
- pain management
- positioning
- activity restrictions

TRANSURETHRAL RESECTION (Prostate, Bladder Tumor)

See also Surgery (General).

Preoperative Period

Knowledge Deficit: (specify)
- examples:
  - postoperative procedures
    - foley catheter
    - murphy irrigation
    - nephrostomy/pyelostomy tubes
  - activity restrictions

Postoperative Period

Potential Complications:
- *Oliguria/anuria*
- *Hemorrhage*
- *Perforated bladder (intraoperative)*
- *Infection*
- *Occlusion of drainage devices*

Alteration in Comfort: Pain related to bladder spasms or clots

Potential Sexual Dysfunction related to fear of impotence resulting from surgical intervention

Knowledge Deficit: (specify)
- examples:
  - fluid requirements
  - activity restrictions
  - follow-up care

URINARY DIVERSION (Ileal Conduit, Ureterosigmoidostomy, Cutaneous Ureterostomy, Suprapubic Cystostomy)

See also Surgery (General).

Preoperative Period

Anxiety/Fear related to:
- examples:
  - surgical procedure
  - diagnosis of cancer
  - permanent loss of usual toilet habits
  - effects on relationships
  - management difficulties

Knowledge Deficit: (specify)
  examples:
    procedure
    appliances

Postoperative Period

Potential Complications:

Urinary stasis
Pyelonephritis
Ureteral obstruction
Stomal stenosis
Renal calculi

Potential Impairment of Skin Integrity related to urine irritation around stoma secondary to ill-fitting appliance

Potential Sexual Dysfunction related to effects of surgery on desire or ability to have sexual activity

Grieving: denial, anger, depression related to loss of usual method of toileting and effects on life-style

Potential Disturbance in Self-Concept related to effects of loss of body parts/function on life-style and relationships

Knowledge Deficit: (specify)
  examples:
    condition
    signs and symptoms of complications
    nutritional therapy
    fluid requirements
    stoma care
    odor control
    appliance care
    community services

Obstetric/Gynecologic Conditions

Obstetric Conditions
  Prenatal Period (General)
    Abortion, Induced
    Abortion, Spontaneous
    Cesarean Section (see section on Surgical Procedures)

    - Extrauterine Pregnancy (Ectopic Pregnancy)
    - Hyperemesis Gravidarum
    - Toxemia
    - Uterine Bleeding during Pregnancy
      - Placenta Previa
      - Abruptio Placentae
      - Uterine Rupture
      - Nonmalignant lesions
      - Hydatidiform Mole
  - Intrapartum Period (General)
  - Postpartum Period (General)
    - Mastitis (Lactational)
    - Fetal/Newborn Death
  - Concomitant Medical Conditions
    - Cardiac Disease (Prenatal, Postpartum)
    - Diabetes (Prenatal)
    - Diabetes (Postnatal)
- Gynecologic Conditions
  - Endometriosis
  - Reproductive Tract Infections
    - Vaginitis
    - Endometritis
    - Pelvic Cellulitis
    - Peritonitis
  - Surgical Procedures (see section on Surgical Procedures)
    - Dilatation and Curettage (D&C)
    - Hysterectomy
    - Mastectomy

Obstetric Conditions

PRENATAL PERIOD (General)

Alteration in Comfort: nausea/vomiting related to elevated estrogen levels, decreased blood sugar or decreased gastric motility

Alteration in Comfort: heartburn related to pressure on cardiac sphincter from enlarged uterus

Alteration in Bowel Elimination: Constipation related to decreased gastric motility and pressure of uterus on the lower colon

Activity Intolerance related to fatigue and dyspnea secondary to pressure of enlarging uterus on diaphragm and increased blood volume

Potential Alteration in Oral Mucous Membranes related to hyperemic gums secondary to estrogen and progesterone levels

Fear related to the possibility of having an imperfect baby

Potential for Infection: vaginal related to increased vaginal secretions secondary to hormonal changes

Potential for Injury related to syncope/hypotension secondary to peripheral venous pooling

Alteration in Comfort: headaches related to increased blood volume

Alteration in Comfort: hemorrhoids related to Constipation and increased pressure of the enlarging uterus

Potential Disturbance in Self-Concept related to the effects of pregnancy on bio–psycho–social patterns

Potential Alteration in Parenting (mother, father) related to

examples:

- knowledge deficit
- unwanted pregnancy
- powerlessness
- feelings of incompetency

Knowledge Deficit: (Specify)

examples:

- effects of pregnancy on
  - body systems
    - cardiovascular
    - integumentary
    - gastrointestinal
    - urinary
    - pulmonary
    - musculoskeletal
  - psychosocial domain
  - sexuality/sexual function
  - family unit
    - spouse
    - children
  - fetal growth and development
  - nutritional requirements

hazards of
- smoking
- excessive alcohol intake
- drug abuse
- excessive caffeine intake
- excessive weight gain

signs and symptoms of complications:
- vaginal bleeding
- cramping
- gestational diabetes
- excessive edema
- pre-eclampsia

preparation for child birth
- classes
- printed references

ABORTION, INDUCED

Preprocedure Period

Knowledge Deficit: (specify)
examples:
- options available
- procedure
- postprocedure care
- normalcy of emotions

Postprocedure Period

Potential Ineffective Individual Coping: depression related to unresolved emotional responses (guilt) to societal, moral, religious, and familial negative influences

Potential Alteration in Family Processes related to the effects of the abortion on relationships (disagreement regarding decisions, previous conflicts [personal, marital] or adolescent identity problems)

Knowledge Deficit: (specify)
examples:
- self-care
  - hygiene
  - breast care
- nutritional needs
- expected bleeding, cramping
- signs and symptoms of complications
- resumption of sexual activity
- contraception

sex education as indicated
comfort measures
expected emotional responses
follow-up appointment
community resources

ABORTION, SPONTANEOUS

Fear related to the possibility of subsequent future abortions
Grieving: denial, anger, depression related to the loss of pregnancy

EXTRAUTERINE PREGNANCY

(Ectopic Pregnancy)

Potential Complications:
Hemorrhage
Shock
Infection
Sepsis

Grieving related to loss of fetus
Fear related to possibility of not being able to carry subsequent pregnancies
Alteration in Comfort: Pain related to rupture of the fallopian tube

HYPEREMESIS GRAVIDARUM

Potential Complications:
Dehydration
Negative nitrogen balance

Potential Alteration in Nutrition: Less than Body Requirements related to vomiting
Anxiety related to ambivalent feeling concerning pregnancy and parenthood

TOXEMIA

See also Prenatal Period.
See also Postpartum Period.

Potential Complications:
Hypertension
Seizures
Coma
Renal failure
Proteinuria
Visual disturbances
Cerebral edema
Fetal compromise

Activity Intolerance related to compromised oxygen supply
Anxiety/Fear related to the effects of condition on self, pregnancy, and infant
Potential Impairment of Skin Integrity related to generalized edema
Fluid Volume Excess: edema related to retention of water and impairment in sodium excretion secondary to impaired renal function
Potential for Injury related to vertigo, visual disturbances, or seizures
Knowledge Deficit: (specify)
examples:
- dietary restrictions
- signs and symptoms of complications
- conservation of energy
- pharmacologic therapy
- comfort measures (headaches, backaches)

UTERINE BLEEDING DURING PREGNANCY
(Placenta Previa, Abruptio Placentae, Uterine Rupture, Nonmalignant Lesions, Hydatidiform mole)

See also Postpartum Period.
Potential Complications:
- *Hemorrhage*
- *Shock*
- *Disseminated intravascular coagulation*
- *Renal failure*
- *Fetal death*
- *Anemia*
- *Sepsis*

Anxiety/Fear related to the effects of bleeding on pregnancy and on infant
Activity Intolerance related to the increased bleeding in response to activity
Grieving related to anticipated loss of pregnancy and loss of expected child
Fear related to possibility of subsequent future pregnancy complications

INTRAPARTUM PERIOD (General)

Potential Complications:
- *Hemorrhage (placenta previa, abruptio placentae)*
- *Fetal distress*
- *Hypertension*
- *Uterine rupture*

Alteration in Comfort related to uterine contractions during labor

Fear related to unpredictability of uterine contractions and possibility of having an impaired baby

Knowledge Deficit:
- examples:
  - relaxation/breathing exercises
  - positioning
  - procedures
    - preparations (bowel, skin)
    - frequent assessments
    - anesthesia (regional, inhalation)

POSTPARTUM PERIOD (General; Mastitis [Lactational]; Fetal/Newborn Death)

General Postpartum Period

Potential Complications:

- *Hemorrhage*
- *Uterine atony*
- *Lacerations*
- *Hematomas*
- *Retained placental fragments*
- *Urinary retention*

Potential for Infection: vaginal, perineal related to bacterial invasion secondary to trauma during labor and delivery and episiotomy

Potential for Infection: breast related to milk production, and trauma during breastfeeding

Alteration in Comfort: Pain related to
- examples:
  - trauma to perineum during labor and delivery
  - hemorrhoids
  - engorged breasts
  - involution of uterus

Potential Alteration in Bowel Elimination: Constipation related to decreased intestinal peristalsis (post delivery) and decreased activity

Potential Alteration in Parenting related to
- examples:
  - inexperience
  - feelings of incompetency
  - powerlessness
  - unwanted child
  - disappointment with child
  - lack of role models

Potential Alteration in Patterns of Urinary Elimination: stress incontinence related to tissue trauma during delivery
Potential Sleep Rest Disturbance related to maternity department's routines and demands of newborn
Potential Disturbance in Self-Concept related to body changes that persist postdelivery (skin, weight and change in life-style)
Knowledge Deficit: (specify)
- examples:
  - postpartum routines
  - hygiene
    - breast
    - perineum
  - exercises
  - sexual counseling (contraception)
  - nutritional requirements
  - infant care
  - stresses of parenthood
  - adaptation of fathers
  - sibling relationships
  - parent/infant bonding
  - postpartum emotional responses
  - sleep/rest requirements
  - household management
  - community resources
  - management of discomforts
    - breast
    - perineum
  - social requirements
    - mother
    - couple
  - signs and symptoms of complications

Mastitis *(Lactational)*

Potential Complications:
- *abscess*

Alteration in Comfort: Pain related to inflammation of breast tissue
Knowledge Deficit: (specify)
- examples:
  - need for breast support
  - breast hygiene

breast feeding restrictions
signs and symptoms of abscess formation

Fetal/Newborn Death

Alteration in Family Processes related to emotional trauma of loss on each family member
Grieving: anger, denial, depression related to loss of child
Fear related to the possibility of future fetal deaths

CONCOMITANT MEDICAL CONDITIONS

(Cardiac Disease [prenatal, postpartum], Diabetes [prenatal, postpartum])

Cardiac Disease

See also Cardiac Disorders.
See also Prenatal Period.
See also Postpartum Period.
Potential Complications:
Congestive heart failure
Toxemia
Eclampsia
Valvular damage
Anxiety/Fear related to the effects of condition on self, pregnancy, and infant
Activity Intolerance related to increased metabolic requirements (pregnancy) in the presence of compromised cardiac function
Impaired Home Maintenance Management related to impaired ability to perform role responsibilities during and after pregnancy
Potential Alteration in Family Processes related to the disruption of activity restrictions and fears on life-style
Knowledge Deficit: (specify)
examples:
dietary requirements (iron, protein)
prevention of infection
conservation of energy
signs and symptoms of complications
community resources

Diabetes (Prenatal)

See also Prenatal Period.
See also Diabetes Mellitus.
See also Postpartum Period.

Potential Complications:
Hypo- /hyperglycemia
Hydramnios
Acidosis
Toxemia

Potential Impairment in Skin Integrity related to excessive skin stretching secondary to hydramnios
Potential for Infection: vaginal related to monilial infection
Alteration in Comfort: headaches related to cerebral edema or hyperirritability
Knowledge Deficit: (specify)
examples:
effects of pregnancy on diabetes
effects of diabetes on pregnancy
nutritional requirements
insulin requirements
signs and symptoms of complications
frequent blood/urine samples

Diabetes (Postpartum)

See also Postpartum Period (General).
Potential Complications:
Hypoglycemia
Hyperglycemia
Toxemia
Eclampsia
Hemorrhage (secondary to uterine atony from excessive amniotic fluid)

Anxiety related to separation from infant secondary to the need for special care needs of infant
Potential for Infection: perineal area related to depleted host defenses and depressed leukocytic phagocytosis secondary to hyperglycemia
Knowledge Deficit: (specify)
examples:
risks of future pregnancies
birth control methods
types
contraindicated
special care requirements for infant

Gynecologic Conditions

ENDOMETRIOSIS

Potential Complications:
Hypermenorrhea
Polymenorrhea

Alteration in Comfort: Pain related to response of displaced endometrial tissue (abdominal, peritoneal) to cyclic ovarian hormonal stimulation
Sexual Dysfunction related to painful intercourse or infertility
Anxiety/Fear related to unpredictable nature of the disease
Knowledge Deficit: (specify)
examples:
condition
myths
pharmacologic therapy
pregnancy potential

REPRODUCTIVE TRACT INFECTIONS (Vaginitis, Endometritis, Pelvic Cellulitis, Peritonitis)

Potential Complications:
Septicemia
Abscess formation
Pneumonia
Pulmonary embolism
Alteration in Comfort: Pain, chills related to infectious process
Potential Fluid Volume Deficit related to inadequate intake, fatigue, pain, and fluid losses secondary to elevated temperature
Potential Ineffective Individual Coping: depression related to the chronicity of the condition and the lack of definitive diagnosis/treatment
Knowledge Deficit: (specify)
examples:
condition
nutritional requirements
signs and symptoms of reoccurrence/ complications
sleep/rest requirements

Neonatal Conditions

Neonate (Normal)
Neonate (Premature)

- Neonate (Postmature)
  - Small for Gestational Age (SGA)
  - Large for Gestational Age (LGA)
- Neonate with Special Problems
  - Congenital Infections
    - Cytomegalovirus
    - Rubella
    - Toxoplasmosis
    - Syphilis
    - Herpes
  - Diabetic Mother
  - High-Risk Neonates
  - Family of The High-Risk Neonate
  - Hyperbilirubinemia
    - Rh Incompatibility
    - ABO Incompatibility
  - Narcotic-Addicted Mother
  - Respiratory Distress Syndrome
  - Sepsis (Septicemia)

NEONATE, NORMAL

Potential Complications:
Hypothermia
Hypoglycemia
Hyperbilirubinemia
Bradycardia

Potential for Infection (nosocomial) related to
vulnerability of infant
lack of normal flora
environmental hazards
personnel
other newborns
parents
open wounds
umbilical cord
circumcision

Potential Alteration in Respiratory Function related to oropharynx secretions

Potential Impairment of Skin Integrity related to susceptibility to nosocomial infection and lack of normal skin flora

Potential Alteration in Tissue Perfusion related to hypothermia

Knowledge Deficit (see Postpartum Period)

NEONATE, PREMATURE

See also Family of High Risk Newborns.
Potential Complications:

- *Cold stress*
- *Apnea*
- *Bradycardia*
- *Hypoglycemia*
- *Acidosis*
- *Hypocalcemia*
- *Sepsis*
- *Seizures*
- *Pneumonia*
- *Hyperbilirubinemia*

Potential Alteration in Nutrition: Less than Body Requirements related to diminished sucking

Potential Alteration in Bowel Elimination: Constipation related to decreased intestinal motility and immobility

Potential Alteration in Respiratory Function related to immobility and increased secretions

Potential for Infection (nosocomial) related to:
- vulnerability of infant
- lack of normal flora
- environmental hazards
- personnel
- other newborns
- parents
- open wounds
  - umbilical cord
  - circumcision

Potential Impairment of Skin Integrity related to susceptibility to nosocomial infection (lack of normal skin flora)

NEONATE, POSTMATURE (Small for Gestation Age [SGA] or Large for Gestation Age [LGA])

Potential Complications:
- Asphyxia at birth
- Meconium aspiration
- Hypoglycemia
- Polycythemia (SGA)
- Edema
  - Generalized
  - Cerebral
- Central nervous system depression
- Renal tubular necrosis

Impaired intestinal absorption
Birth injuries (LGA)
Potential Impairment of Skin Integrity related to absence of protective vernix and prolonged exposure to amniotic fluid (LGA)
Potential Alteration in Nutrition: Less than Body Requirements related to swallowing difficulties
Potential Alteration in Tissue Perfusion related to hypothermia

NEONATE WITH SPECIAL PROBLEM

(Congenital Infections—Cytomegalovirus [CMV], Rubella, Toxoplasmosis, Syphilis, Herpes)

See also High-Risk Neonates.
See also Family of High-Risk Neonate.
See also Developmental Problems/Needs under Pediatric Disorders.

Potential Complications:

Hyperbilirubinemia
Hepatosplenomegaly
Anemia
Hydrocephalus
Microcephaly
Mental retardation
Congenital heart disease (rubella)
Cataracts (rubella)
Retinitis
Thrombocytopenia purpura (rubella)
Sensorimotor deafness (CMV)
Periostitis (syphilis)
Seizures

Potential for Infection to others related to contagious nature of the organism
Potential for Injury related to uncontrolled tonic/clonic movements
Potential Alteration in Nutrition: Less than Body Requirements, related to poor sucking reflex

DIABETIC MOTHER

See also Neonate (normal).
See also Families of High-Risk Neonates.

Potential Complications:

Hypoglycemia
Hypocalcemia
Polycythemia
Hyperbilirubinemia
Sepsis
Acidosis
Birth injury (macrosomia)
Hyaline membrane disease (if premature)

respiratory distress syndrome — *venous thrombosis*

Potential Fluid Volume Deficit related to increased urinary excretion and osmotic diuresis

HIGH-RISK NEONATES

See also Family of High-Risk Neonate.

Potential Complications:

Anoxia — *Seizures*
Shock — *Hypotension*
Respiratory distress — *Septicemia*

Alteration in Comfort related to abdominal distention

Potential Alteration in Nutrition: Less than Body Requirements related to poor sucking reflex secondary to (specify)

Potential for Injury related to uncontrolled tonic/clonic movements or hyperirritability

Potential for Infection (nosocomial) related to
- vulnerability of infant
- lack of normal flora
- environmental hazards
  - personnel
  - other newborns
  - parents
- open wounds
  - umbilical cord
  - circumcision

Potential Alteration in Respiratory Function related to oropharynx secretions

Potential Impairment of Skin Integrity related to susceptibility to nosocomial infection secondary to lack of normal skin flora

Potential Alteration in Tissue Perfusion related to hypothermia

FAMILY OF THE HIGH-RISK NEONATE

Grieving related to the realization of present or future loss for themselves and/or child

Alteration in Family Processes related to the effect of extended hospitalization on family (role responsibilities, financial)

Anxiety related to the unpredictable prognosis of child

Potential Alteration in Parenting related to inadequate bonding secondary to parental child separation or failure to accept impaired child

Ineffective Individual Coping: depression, guilt related to perceived parental role failure

HYPERBILIRUBINEMIA (Rh incompatibility, ABO incompatibility)

See also Family of High-Risk Neonate.
See also Neonate (Normal).

Potential Complications:

- *Anemia*
- *Jaundice*
- *Kernicterus*
- *Hepatosplenomegaly*
- *Hydrops fetalis (cardiac failure, hypoxia, anasarca, pericardial, pleural and peritoneal effusions)*
- *Renal failure (phototherapy complications, hyperthermia/hypothermia, dehydration, priapism, "bronze-baby" syndrome)*

Potential for Injury: ophthalmic related to exposure to phototherapy light and continuous wearing of eye pads

Potential Impairment of Skin Integrity related to diarrhea, urinary excretions of bilirubin, and exposure to phototherapy light

NARCOTIC-ADDICTED MOTHER

See also Family of High-Risk Neonate.
See also Neonate (Normal).
See also Substance Abuse for Mother.

Potential Complications:

- *Hyperirritability/seizures*
- *Withdrawal*
- *Hypocalcemia*
- *Hypoglycemia*
- *Sepsis*
- *Dehydration*
- *Electrolyte imbalances*
- *Aspiration*

Potential Alteration in Nutrition: Less than Body Requirements related to uncoordinated and ineffective sucking and swallowing reflexes

Potential Impairment of Skin Integrity related to generalized diaphoresis and marked rigidity

Alteration in Bowel Elimination: Diarrhea related to increased peristalsis secondary to hyperirritability
Sleep-Rest Disturbance related to hyperirritability
Potential for Injury: blisters related to frantic sucking of fists
Potential for Injury related to uncontrolled tremors or tonic/clonic movements
Sensory Perceptual Alterations related to hypersensitivity to environmental stimuli

RESPIRATORY DISTRESS SYNDROME

See also High-Risk Neonates.
See also Mechanical Ventilation.
Potential Complications:

Hypoxia
Atelectasis
Acidosis
Sepsis
Hyperthermia

Activity Intolerance related to insufficient oxygenation of tissues secondary to impaired respirations
Potential for Infection (nosocomial) related to vulnerability of infant, lack of normal flora, environmental hazards (personnel, other newborns, parents), and open wounds (umbilical cord, circumcision)
Potential Impairment of Skin Integrity related to Susceptibility to nosocomial infection and Lack of normal skin flora

SEPSIS (Septicemia)

See also Newborn.
See also Family of High-Risk Neonate.
Potential Complications:

Anemia
Respiratory distress
Hypothermia/hyperthermia
Hypotension
Edema
Seizures
Hepatosplenomegaly
Hemorrhage
Jaundice
Meningitis
Pyarthrosis

Potential Impairment of Skin Integrity related to edema and immobility
Alteration in Nutrition: Less than Body Requirements related to poor sucking reflex

Alteration in Bowel Elimination: Diarrhea related to intestinal irritation secondary to infecting organism
Potential for Injury related to uncontrolled tonic/clonic movements
Potential for Injury: ecchymosis related to hematopoietic insufficiency

Pediatric/Adolescent Disorders*

- Developmental Problems/Needs related to
  - Chronic Illness
  - Permanent Disability
  - Multiple Handicaps
  - Developmental Disability (Mental/Physical)
  - Life-Threatening Illness
- Asthma
- Celiac Disease
- Cerebral Palsy
- Child Abuse
  - Battered Child Syndrome
  - Child Neglect
- Cleft Lip and Palate
- Communicable Diseases
- Convulsive Disorders
- Cystic Fibrosis
- Down's Syndrome
- Failure to Thrive (Nonorganic)
- Glomerular Disorders
  - Glomerulonephritis (Acute, Chronic)
  - Nephrotic Syndrome (Congenital, Secondary, Idiopathic)

* For additional pediatric medical diagnoses, see the adult diagnoses and also Developmental Problems/Needs; for example:

Diabetes mellitus
Anorexia nervosa (psychiatric disorders)
Spinal cord injury
Head trauma
Neoplastic disorders
Fractures
Congestive heart failure
Pneumonia

Hemophilia
Infectious Mononucleosis (Adolescent)
Legg-Calve-Perthes Disease
Leukemia
Meningitis (Bacterial)
Meningomyelocele
Mental Retardation
Muscular Dystrophy (Duchenne's)
Obesity
Osteomyelitis
Parasitic Disorders
Poisoning
Respiratory Tract Infections (Lower)
Rheumatic Fever
Rheumatoid Arthritis (Juvenile)
Reye's Syndrome
Scoliosis
Sickle Cell Anemia
Tonsillitis
Wilms' Tumor

DEVELOPMENTAL PROBLEMS/NEEDS RELATED TO CHRONIC ILLNESS

Examples: permanent disability
multiple handicaps
developmental disability (mental/physical)
life-threatening illness

Grieving (parental): denial, anger, depression related to the anticipated losses secondary to the condition
Alteration in Family Processes related to the adjustment requirements for the situation
examples:
- time
- energy
  - emotional
  - physical
- financial
- physical care

Potential Impaired Home Maintenance Management related to inadequate resources, housing or impaired caregiver(s)

Potential Social Isolation (child/family) related to the disability and the requirements of the caregiver(s)
Potential Alteration in Parenting related to abuse, rejection, overprotection secondary to inadequate resources or coping mechanisms
Anxiety (parental) related to illness, health-care interventions and parental/child separation
Self-Care Deficit: (specify) related to illness limitations or hospitalization
Potential Disturbance in Self-Concept related to impaired ability to achieve developmental tasks secondary to restrictions imposed by disease, disability, or treatments

ASTHMA

See also Developmental Problems/Needs.
Potential Complications:
- *Hypoxia*
- *Respiratory acidosis*
- *Corticosteroid therapy*

Ineffective Airway Clearance related to bronchospasm and increased pulmonary secretions
Anxiety related to breathlessness and fear of reoccurrence
Potential Alteration in Respiratory Function related to increased pulmonary secretions
Knowledge Deficit: (specify)
- examples:
  - condition
  - environmental hazards
    - smoking
    - allergens
    - weather
  - prevention of infection
  - breathing/relaxation exercises
  - signs and symptoms of complications
  - pharmacologic therapy
  - fluid requirements
  - Behavioral modification
    - daily diary recording

CELIAC DISEASE

See also Developmental Problems/Needs.

Potential Complications:
- *Severe malnutrition/ dehydration*
- *Anemia*
- *Altered blood coagulation*
- *Osteoporosis*
- *Electrolyte imbalances*
- *Metabolic acidosis*
- *Shock*
- *Delayed growth*

Potential Alteration in Nutrition: Less than Body Requirements related to malabsorption, dietary restrictions and anorexia

Alteration in Bowel Elimination: diarrhea/steatorrhea related to decreased absorption in small intestines secondary to damaged villi resulting from toxins from undigested gliadin

Potential Fluid Volume Deficit related to fluid loss in diarrhea

Knowledge Deficit: (specify)

examples:
- dietary management
  - restrictions
  - vitamin
  - protein
  - carbohydrate requirements

CEREBRAL PALSY*

See also Developmental Problems/Needs.

Potential Complications:
- *Contractures*
- *Seizures*
- *Respiratory infections*

Potential for Injury related to inability to control movements

Potential Alteration in Nutrition: Less than Body Requirements related to sucking difficulties (infant) and dysphagia

Self-Care Deficit (specify) related to sensory/motor impairments

Sensory Perceptual Alterations: Visual, Auditory, Tactile, related to sensory impairment

* Because disabilities associated with cerebral palsy can be varied (hemiparesis, quadriparesis, diplegia, monoplegeia, triplegia, paraplegia), the nurse will have to clearly specify the child's limitations in the diagnostic statements.

Impaired Verbal Communication related to impaired ability to speak words related to facial muscle involvement
Potential Fluid Volume Deficit related to difficulty obtaining or swallowing liquids
Potential Diversional Activity Deficit related to the effects of limitations on ability to participate in recreational activities
Knowledge Deficit: (specify)
examples:
- disease
- pharmacologic regime
- activity program
- education
- community services
- orthopedic appliances

CHILD ABUSE (Battered Child Syndrome; Child Neglect)

See also Fractures, Burns.
See also Failure to Thrive.
Potential Complications:
- *Trauma (fractures, burns, lacerations)*
- *Behavioral disorders (withdrawal, aggression)*
- *Failure to thrive*
- *Malnutrition*
- *Vandalism*
- *Drug or alcohol addiction (older child)*
- *Venereal disease*
- *Pregnancy in young adolescent*

Alteration in Parenting related to presence of factors that contribute to child abuse:
examples:
- lack of or unavailability of the extended family
- economic conditions
  - inflation
  - unemployment
- lack of role model as a child
- high-risk children
  - unwanted
  - of undesired sex or appearance
  - physically or mentally handicapped
  - hyperactive
  - terminally ill

high-risk parents
- single
- adolescent
- emotionally disturbed
- alcoholic
- drug addicted
- physically ill

Ineffective Individual Coping (child abuser) related to
examples:
- history of abuse by own parents and lack of warmth and affection from them
- social isolation (few friends or outlets for tensions)
- marked lack of self-esteem, with low tolerance for criticism
- emotional immaturity and dependency
- distrust of others
- inability to admit the need for help
- high expectations for/of child (perceiving child as a source of emotional gratification)
- unrealistic desire for the child to give them pleasure

Ineffective Individual Coping (nonabusing parent) related to passive and compliant response to abuse

Fear related to possibility of placement in a shelter or foster home

Anxiety/Fear (parental) related to responses of others guilt, possible loss of child, and criminal prosecution

Potential Alteration in Nutrition: Less than Body Requirements related to inadequate intake secondary to lack of knowledge or neglect

Knowledge Deficit, (specify)
examples:
- parenting skills
  - discipline
  - expectations
- constructive stress management
- signs and symptoms of abuse
- high-risk groups
  - parents
  - child
- child protection laws
- community services
  - hot-lines
  - counselling

CLEFT LIP AND PALATE

See also Developmental Problems/Needs.
See also Surgery (General).

Preoperative Period

Potential Alteration in Nutrition: Less than Body Requirements related to inability to suck secondary to cleft lip

Postoperative Period

Potential Complications:

Aspiration
Failure to thrive
Respiratory distress

Impaired Physical Mobility related to restricted activity secondary to the use of restraints
Potential Impaired Verbal Communication related to impaired muscle development, insufficient palate function, faulty dentation, or hearing loss
Knowledge Deficit: (specify)
examples:
condition
feeding and suctioning techniques
surgical site care
risks for otis media (dental/oral problems)
referral to speech therapist

COMMUNICABLE DISEASES

See also Developmental Problems/Needs.

Alteration in Comfort related to fatigue, malaise, sore throat, and elevated temperature
Potential for Infection to others related to contagious agents
Potential Fluid Volume Deficit related to increased fluid loss secondary to elevated temperature or insufficient oral intake secondary to malaise
Impairment of Skin Integrity related to pruritus
Sensory Perceptual Alterations: Visual related to photophobia (rubeola)
Potential Alteration in Nutrition: Less than Body Requirements related to anorexia and sore throat or pain on chewing (mumps)

Potential Ineffective Airway Clearance related to increased mucous production (whooping cough)
Knowledge Deficit: (specify)
examples:
condition
transmission
prevention
immunizations
skin care

CONVULSIVE DISORDERS

See also Developmental Problems/Needs.
See also Mental Retardation if indicated.
Potential Complications:
Respiratory arrest
Hypoxia
Potential for Injury related to uncontrolled movements seizure activity
Anxiety related to embarassment and fear of seizure episodes
Potential Ineffective Individual Coping: aggression related to restrictions, parental overprotection, and parental indulgence
Knowledge Deficit: (specify)
examples:
condition/cause
pharmacologic therapy
treatment during seizures
seizure precautions
environmental hazards
water
driving
heights

CYSTIC FIBROSIS

See also Developmental Problems/Needs.
Potential Complications:
Infection
Bronchopneumonia, atelectasis
Paralytic ileus
Ineffective Airway Clearance related to mucopurulent secretions

Potential Alteration in Nutrition: Less than Body
Requirements, related to the need for increased calories and protein secondary to impaired intestinal absorption, loss of fat, and fat soluable vitamins in stools

Alteration in Bowel Elimination: Constipation/Diarrhea related to excessive or insufficient pancreatic enzyme replacement

Activity Intolerance related to dyspnea secondary to mucopurulent secretions

Knowledge Deficit: (specify)

examples:
- condition (genetic transmission)
- risk for infection
- pharmacological therapy
  - side effects
  - ototoxicity
  - renal toxicity
- equipment
  - oxygen
  - nebulization
- nutritional therapy
- salt replacement requirements
- breathing exercises
- postural drainage
- exercise program
- community resources (Cystic Fibrosis Foundation)

DOWN'S SYNDROME

See also Developmental Problems/Needs.
See also Mental Retardation if indicated.

Potential Alteration in Respiratory Function related to decreased respiratory expansion secondary to decreased muscle tone, inadequate mucous drainage, and mouth breathing

Potential Impairment of Skin Integrity related to rough, dry skin surface and flaccid extremities

Potential Alteration in Bowel Elimination: Constipation related to decreased gastric motility

Alteration in Nutrition: Less than Body Requirements (infant) related to sucking difficulties secondary to large protruding tongue

Potential Alteration in Nutrition: Greater than Body Requirements related to increased caloric consumption secondary to boredom in the presence of limited physical activity

Self-Care Deficits: (specify) related to physical limitations

Knowledge Deficit: (specify)

examples:
- condition
- home care
- education
- community services

FAILURE TO THRIVE (Nonorganic)

See also Developmental Problems/Needs.

Potential Complications:
- *Metabolic dysfunction*
- *Dehydration*

Ineffective Individual Coping (caregiver) related to failure to respond to child's needs (emotional/physical) secondary to caregiver's emotional problems

Alteration in Nutrition: Less than Body Requirements related to inadequate intake secondary to the lack of emotional and sensory stimulation or lack of knowledge of caregiver

Sensory Perceptual Alterations related to a history of insufficient sensory input from primary caregiver

Sleep Pattern Disturbance related to anxiety and apprehension secondary to parental deprivation

Alteration in Parenting related to

examples:
- lack of knowledge of parenting skills
- impaired caregiver
- impaired child
- lack of support system
- lack of role model
- relationship problems
- unrealistic expectations for child
- unmet psychological needs

Impaired Home Maintenance Management related to difficulty of caretaker to maintain a safe home environment

Knowledge Deficit: (specify)

examples:
- growth and development requirements
- feeding guidelines
- risk for child abuse
- parenting skills
- community agencies

GLOMERULAR DISORDERS (Glomerulonephritis: Acute, Chronic; Nephrotic Syndrome: Congenital, Secondary, Idiopathic)

See also Developmental Problems/Needs.
See also Corticosteroid Therapy.
Potential Complications:
- *Anasarca (generalized edema)*
- *Hypertension*
- *Azotemia*
- *Septicemia*
- *Malnutrition*
- *Ascites*
- *Pleural effusion*
- *Hypoalbuminemia*

Potential for Infection related to increased susceptibility during edematous phase and lowered resistance secondary to corticosteroid therapy

Potential Impairment of Skin Integrity related to
- examples:
  - immobility
  - lowered resistance
  - edema
  - frequent application of collection bags

Alteration in Nutrition: Less than Body Requirements related to dietary restrictions, anorexia secondary to fatigue, malaise, and pressure on abdominal structures (edema)

Activity Intolerance related to fatigue

Diversional Activity Deficit related to hospitalization and impaired ability to perform usual activities

Knowledge Deficit: (specify)
- examples:
  - condition
  - etiology
  - course
- treatments
- signs and symptoms of complications
- pharmacologic therapy
- nutritional/fluid requirements
- prevention of infection
- home care
  - diet
  - urine testing
- follow-up care
- community services

HEMOPHILIA

See also Developmental Problems/Needs.
Potential Complications:
Hemorrhage
Potential for Injury related to increased risk of hemorrhage secondary to clotting factor deficiencies
Alteration in Comfort: Pain related to joint swelling and limitations secondary to hemarthrosis
Potential Impaired Physical Mobility related to joint swelling and limitations secondary to hemarthrosis
Potential Alteration in Oral Mucous Membranes related to trauma from coarse food and insufficient dental hygiene
Knowledge Deficit: (specify)
examples:
condition
contraindications (*e.g.*, aspirin)
genetic transmission
environmental hazards
emergency treatment to control bleeding

INFECTIOUS MONONUCLEOSIS (Adolescent)

Potential Complications:
Enlarged spleen
Hepatic dysfunction
Activity Intolerance related to fatigue secondary to infectious process
Alteration in Comfort: Pain related to sore throat and headaches
Alteration in Health Maintenance related to the need for nutritional counseling and sleep requirements
Potential Alteration in Nutrition: Less than Body Requirements related to sore throat and malaise
Grieving: anger and depression related to the restrictions of the disease and treatments on life-style
Knowledge Deficit: (specify)
examples:
condition
communicable nature
diet therapy
risks of alcohol ingestion (with hepatic dysfunction)

- signs and symptoms of complications
  - hepatic
  - splenic
  - neurologic
  - hematologic
- activity restrictions

LEGG–CALVÉ–PERTHES DISEASE

See also Developmental Problems/Needs.

Potential Complications:
- *permanent deformed femoral head*

Alteration in Comfort: Pain related to joint dysfunction

Impaired Physical Mobility related to non-weight-bearing regime or immobilization devices (casts, braces)

Potential Impairment of Skin Integrity related to immobilization devices (casts, braces)

Self Care Deficits: (specify) related to pain and immobilization devices

Knowledge Deficit: (specify)
- examples:
  - disease
  - weight-bearing restrictions
  - application/maintenance of devices
  - pain management at home

LEUKEMIA

See also Chemotherapy.

See also Radiation Therapy

See also Cancer (GENERAL).

See also Developmental Problems/Needs.

Potential Complications:
- *Hepatosplenomegaly*
- *Increased intracranial edema*
- *Metastasis (brain, lungs, kidneys, gastrointestinal tract, spleen, liver)*
- *Hypermetabolism*
- *Hemorrhage*
- *Dehydration*
- *Myclosupression*

Potential for Infection related to altered immune system secondary to leukemic process and side effects of chemotherapeutic agents

Potential Social Isolation related to the effects of disease and treatments on appearance and the fear of embarassment
Potential Disturbance in Self-Concept related to impaired ability to achieve developmental tasks secondary to limitations of disease and treatments

MENINGITIS (Bacterial)

See also Developmental Problems/Needs.
Potential Complications:
Peripheral circulatory collapse
Diffuse intravascular coagulation
Increased intracranial pressure/hydrocephalus
Visual/auditory nerve palsies
Paresis (hemi-, quadri-)
Subdural effusions
Respiratory distress
Seizures
Fluid/electrolyte imbalances
Potential for Injury related to seizure activity secondary to infectious process
Alteration in Comfort related to nuchal rigity, muscle aches, and immobility
Sensory Perceptual Alteration: Visual, Auditory related to increased sensitivity to external stimuli secondary to infectious process
Impaired Physical Mobility related to intravenous infusion, nuchal rigidity, and restraining devices
Potential Impairment of Skin Integrity related to immobility
Knowledge Deficit: (specify)
examples:
condition
antibiotic therapy
diagnostic procedures

MENINGOMYELOCELE

See also Developmental Problems/Needs.
Potential Complications:
Hydrocephalus/shunt infections
Increased intracranial pressure
Urinary tract infections

Potential for Infection related to vulnerability of meningomyelocele sac
Potential Impairment of Skin Integrity related to sensorimotor impairments and orthopedic appliances
Self-Care Deficit: (specify) related to sensorimotor impairments
Potential for Injury: fractures, membrane tears related to pathological condition
Impaired Physical Mobility related to lower limb impairments
Grieving (parental) related to the birth of infant with deficits
Alteration in Patterns of Urinary Elimination: incontinence related to sensorimotor impairments
Knowledge Deficit: (specify)
examples:
condition
home care
orthopedic appliances
self-catheterization
activity program
community services

MENTAL RETARDATION

See Developmental Problems/Needs.
Self-Care Deficit: (specify) related to sensorimotor deficits
Impaired Verbal Communication related to impaired receptive skills or impaired expressive skills
Potential Social Isolation (family, child) related to fear and embarrassment of child's behavior/appearance
Knowledge Deficits: (specify)
examples:
condition
child's potential
home care
community services
education

MUSCULAR DYSTROPHY (Duchenne's)

See also Developmental Problems/Needs.
Potential Complications:
Contractures
Seizures
Respiratory infections
Metabolic failure
Potential for Injury related to inability to control movements

Potential Alteration in Nutrition: Less than Body Requirements related to sucking difficulties (infant) and dysphagia

Self-Care Deficits: (specify) related to sensorimotor impairments

Sensory Perceptual Alterations: visual, auditory, tactile, related to sensory impairment

Impaired Verbal Communication related to impaired ability to speak words secondary to facial muscle involvement

Impaired Physical Mobility related to muscle weakness

Potential Alteration in Nutrition: More than Body Requirements, related to increased caloric consumption secondary to boredom in the presence of decreased metabolic needs secondary to limited physical activity

Grieving (parental) related to progressive terminal nature of the disease

Potential Fluid Volume Deficit related to difficulty obtaining or swallowing liquids

Potential Diversional Activity Deficit related to the effects of limitations on the ability to participate in recreational activities

Knowledge Deficit: (specify)
examples:
disease
pharmacologic regime
activity program
education
community services

OBESITY

See also Developmental Problems/Needs.

Ineffective Individual Coping related to increased food consumption in response to stressors

Alteration in Health Maintenance related to the need for
Exercise program
Nutrition counseling
Behavioral modification

Disturbance in Self-Concept related to feelings of self-degradation and the response of others (peers, family, others) to his/her obesity

Alteration in Family Processes related to responses to and the effects of weight loss therapy on the parent/child relationship

Potential Impaired Social Interaction related to an inability to initiate and maintain relationships secondary to feelings of embarassment and negative responses of others

Knowledge Deficit: (specify)

examples:

- condition
  - etiology
  - course
  - risks
- therapies available
- destructive versus constructive eating patterns
- self-help groups

OSTEOMYELITIS

See also Developmental Problems/Needs.

Potential Complications:

Pathological fractures

Infective emboli

Side effects of antibiotic therapy (hematologic, renal, hepatic)

Alteration in Comfort related to swelling, hyperthermia, and the infectious process of the bone

Diversional Activity Deficit related to impaired mobility and long-term hospitalization

Potential Alteration in Nutrition: Less than Body Requirements, related to anorexia secondary to infectious process

Potential Alteration in Bowel Elimination: Constipation related to immobility

Potential Impairment of Skin Integrity related to mechanical irritation of cast/splint

Knowledge Deficit: (specify)

examples:

- condition
- wound care
- activity restrictions
- signs and symptoms of complications
- pharmacologic therapy
- follow-up care

PARASITIC DISORDERS

See also Developmental Problems/Needs.

Potential Alteration in Nutrition: Less than Body Requirements related to anorexia, nausea vomiting, and deprivation of host nutrients by parasites

Impairment of Skin Integrity related to pruritus secondary to emergence of parasites (pinworms) onto perianal skin, lytic necrosis, and tissue digestion

Alteration in Bowel Elimination: Diarrhea related to parasitic irritation to intestinal mucosa

Alteration in Comfort: abdominal pain related to parasitic invasion of small intestines

Knowledge Deficit: (specify)
- examples:
  - condition
  - mode of transmission
  - prevention of reinfection
    - hygiene
    - clothing

POISONING

See also Dialysis if Indicated.
See also Unconscious Individual.
Potential Complications:

- *Respiratory alkalosis*
- *Metabolic acidosis*
- *Hemorrhage*
- *Fluid/electrolyte imbalance*
- *Burns (acid/alkaline)*
- *Aspiration*
- *Blindness*

Alteration in Comfort: hyperpyrexia related to heat production secondary to poisoning (*e.g.* salicylate)

Potential for Injury related to
- examples:
  - tonic/clonic movement
  - bleeding tendencies

Anxiety/Fear related to invasive nature of treatments (gastric lavage, dialysis)

Anxiety (parental) related to uncertainty of situation and feelings of guilt

Potential for Injury related to lack of awareness of environmental hazards

Knowledge Deficit: (specify)
- examples:
  - condition
  - treatments
  - home treatment of accidental poisoning

poison prevention
storage
teaching
poisonous plants
locks

RESPIRATORY TRACT INFECTION (Lower)

See also Developmental Problems/Needs.
See also Adult Pneumonia.
Potential Complications:
Hyperthermia | *Septic shock*
Respiratory insufficiency | *Paralytic ileus*

Alteration in Comfort related to hyperthermia, malaise, and respiratory distress
Potential Alteration in Nutrition: Less than Body Requirements related to anorexia secondary to dyspnea and malaise
Anxiety related to breathlessness and apprehension
Potential Fluid Volume Deficit related to insufficient intake secondary to dyspnea and malaise
Knowledge Deficit: (specify)
examples:
condition
prevention of recurrence
treatment
oxygen
croup tent

RHEUMATIC FEVER

See also Developmental Problems/Needs.
Potential Complications:
Endocarditis

Diversional Activity Deficit related to prescribed bedrest
Alteration in Nutrition: Less than Body Requirements related to anorexia
Alteration in Comfort related to arthralgia
Potential for Injury related to choreic movements
Potential Noncompliance: long-term antibiotic therapy related to the difficulty of maintaining preventive drugs when illness is resolved

Knowledge Deficit: (specify)
examples:
condition
signs and symptoms of complications
long-term antibiotic therapy
prevention of reoccurence
risk factors
(surgery, *e.g.*, dental)

RHEUMATOID ARTHRITIS (Juvenile)

See also Developmental Problems/Needs.
See also Corticosteroid Therapy.
Potential Complications:
Pericarditis
Iridocyclitis
Activity Intolerance related to fatigue and pain
Impaired Physical Mobility related to pain and restricted joint movement
Alteration in Comfort: Pain related to swollen, inflamed joints and restricted movement
Knowledge Deficit: (specify)
examples:
condition
pharmacologic therapy
exercise program
rest versus activity
myths
community resources

REYE'S SYNDROME

See also Unconscious Individual if Indicated.
Potential Complications:
Renal failure
Increased intracranial pressure
Fluid/electrolyte imbalance
Hepatic failure
Shock
Seizures
Coma
Respiratory distress
Diabetes insipidus
Anxiety (parental) related to diagnosis and uncertain prognosis
Potential for Injury related to uncontrolled tonic/clonic movements
Potential for Infection related to invasive monitoring procedures

Alteration in Comfort related to hyperpyrexia and malaise secondary to disease process
Anxiety/Fear related to separation from family, sensory bombardment (ICU, treatments), and unfamiliar experiences
Alteration in Family Process related to
  Examples:
    Critical nature of syndrome
    Hospitalization of child
    Separation of family members
Grieving: anger, denial, guilt, depression related to actual, anticipated, or possible death of child
Potential Impairment of Skin Integrity related to immobility
Knowledge Deficit: (specify)
  examples:
    condition
      etiology
      course
    treatments
    complications

SCOLIOSIS

See also Developmental Problems/Needs.
  Impaired Physical Mobility related to restricted movement secondary to braces
  Potential Impairment of Skin Integrity related to mechanical irritation of brace
  Potential Noncompliance related to chronicity and complexity of treatment regimen
  Potential for Injury: falls related to restricted range of motion
  Knowledge Deficit: (specify)
    examples:
      condition
      treatment
        medical
        surgical
      exercises
      environmental hazards
      care of appliances
      follow-up care
      community services

SICKLE CELL ANEMIA

See also Developmental Problems/Needs if the individual is a child.

Potential Complications:

- *Sickling crisis*
- *Transfusion therapy*
- *Thrombosis and infarction*
- *Cholelithiasis*

Alteration in Tissue Perfusion: Peripheral related to viscous blood and occulsion of microcirculation

Alteration in Comfort: Pain related to viscous blood and tissue hypoxia

Self-Care Deficit (specify) related to pain and immobility of exacerbations

Knowledge Deficit: (specify)

examples:

- hazards
- signs and symptoms of complications
- fluid requirements
- hereditary factors

TONSILLITIS

See also Tonsillectomy if Indicated.

Potential Complications:

- *Otitis media*
- *Rheumatic fever (β-hemolytic streptococci)*

Alteration in Comfort: Pain related to inflammation

Potential Fluid Volume Deficit related to inadequate fluid intake

Knowledge Deficit: (specify)

examples:

- condition
- treatments
  - medical
  - surgical
- nutritional/fluid requirements
- signs and symptoms of complications

WILMS' TUMOR

See also Developmental Problems/Needs.
See also Nephrectomy.
See also Cancer (General).

Potential Complications:

- *metastases to liver, lung, bone, brain*
- *infection*

Potential for Injury related to rupture of tumor capsule secondary to manipulation/palpation of abdomen

Anxiety/Fear (child) related to
- examples:
  - age-related concerns
    - separation
    - strangers
    - pain
  - response of others to visible signs (alopecia)
  - uncertain future

Anxiety/Fear (parental) related to
- examples:
  - unknown prognosis
  - painful procedures
  - treatments (chemotherapy)
  - feelings of inadequacy

Grieving: anger, denial, guilt, depression related to the actual, anticipated, or possible death of child

Spiritual Distress related to the nature of the disease and its possible disturbances on belief systems

Knowledge Deficit: (specify)
- examples:
  - condition
  - prognosis
  - treatments (side-effects)
  - home care
  - nutritional requirements
  - follow-up care
  - community services

Psychiatric Disorders

- Affective Disorders (Depression)
- Anorexia Nervosa
- Anxiety and Adjustment Disorders
  - Phobias
  - Anxiety States
  - Traumatic Stress Disorders
  - Adjustment Reactions
- Bipolar Disorders (Mania)
- Childhood Behavioral Disorders
  - Attention Deficit Disorders
  - Learning Disabilities

Paranoid Disorders
Personality Disorders
Schizophrenic Disorders
Somatoform Disorders
  Somatization
  Hypochondriasis
  Conversion Reactions
Substance Abuse Disorders

AFFECTIVE DISORDERS (Depression)

Self-Care Deficit: grooming related to decreased interest in body, inability to make decisions, and feelings of worthlessness

Ineffective Individual Coping: anger related to internal conflicts (guilt, low self-esteem) or feelings of rejection

Impaired Social Interactions related to alienation from others by constant complaining, ruminations, or loss of pleasure from relationships

Ineffective Individual Coping: excessive physical complaints (without organic etiology) related to inability to express emotional needs directly

Social Isolation related to inability to initiate activities to reduce isolation secondary to low energy levels

Grieving: pathological pattern related to unresolved grief prolonged denial and repression

Disturbance in Self-Concept related to feelings of worthlessness and failure

Ineffective Family Coping related to marital discord and role conflicts secondary to the effects of chronic depression on its members

Powerlessness related to unrealistic negative beliefs about self-worth or abilities

Alterations in Thought Processes: cognitive distortions related to negative cognitive set (overgeneralizing, polarized thinking, selected abstraction, arbitrary inference)

Sexual Dysfunction related to decreased sex drive, loss of interest and pleasure

Diversional Activity Deficit related to a loss of interest or pleasure in usual activities and low energy levels

Impaired Home Maintenance Management related to inability to make decisions or concentrate

Potential for Violence to self related to feelings of hopelessness and loneliness

Sleep Pattern Disturbance related to difficulty in falling asleep or early morning awakening secondary to emotional stress

Alteration in Bowel Elimination: Constipation related to sedentary life-style, insufficient exercise, or inadequate diet

Potential Alteration in Nutrition: More than Body Requirements, related to increased intake versus decrease activity expenditures secondary to boredom and frustrations

Potential Alteration in Nutrition: Less than Body Requirements related to anorexia secondary to emotional stress

Knowledge Deficit: (specify)
- examples:
  - condition
  - behavior modification
  - therapy options
    - pharmacologic
    - electroshock
  - community resources

ANOREXIA NERVOSA

Potential Complications:
- *Anemia*
- *Cardiac arrhythmias*
- *Hypotension*

Alteration in Nutrition: Less than Body Requirements related to anorexia and self-induced vomiting following eating and laxative abuse

Disturbance in Self-Concept related to inaccurate perception of self as obese

Potential Fluid Volume Deficit related to vomiting and excessive weight loss

Sleep Pattern Disturbance related to fears and anxiety concerning weight status

Activity Intolerance related to fatigue secondary to malnutrition

Ineffective Individual Coping related to self-induced vomiting, denial of hunger, and food binges secondary to feelings of loss of control and inaccurate preceptions of body states

Ineffective Family Coping related to marital discord and its effect on family members

Potential Impairment of Skin Integrity related to dry skin secondary to malnourished state

Alteration in Bowel Elimination: Constipation related to insufficient food and fluid intake

Impaired Social Interactions related to inability to form relationships with others or fear of trusting relationships with others

Fear of Sexuality, Maturity related to dissatisfaction with the relationships of others (parents, peers)

ANXIETY AND ADJUSTMENT DISORDERS

(Phobias, Anxiety States, Traumatic Stress Disorders, Adjustment Reactions)

See also Substance Use Disorders if indicated.

Ineffective Individual Coping related to irrational avoidance of objects or situations

Impaired Social Interactions related to effects of behavior and actions on forming and maintaining relationships

Ineffective Individual Coping related to dependency on drugs

Anxiety related to irrational thoughts or guilt

Social Isolation related to irrational fear of social situations

Ineffective Individual Coping related to avoidance of objects or situations secondary to a numbing of responsiveness following a traumatic event

Sleep Pattern Disturbance related to recurrent nightmares

Disturbance in Self Concept related to feelings of guilt

Ineffective Individual Coping related to altered ability to constructively manage stressors secondary to (specify)

examples:

physical illness
marital discord
business crisis
natural disasters
developmental crisis

Knowledge Deficit:
  examples:
    condition
    pharmacologic therapy
    legal system regarding violence

BIPOLAR DISORDER (Mania)

Disturbance in Self-Concept related to exaggerated sense of self-importance and abilities secondary to feelings of inadequacy and inferiority
Impaired Social Interaction related to overt hostility, overconfidence, or manipulation of others
Potential for Violence to Others related to impaired reality testing, impaired judgement or inability to control behavior
Sleep Pattern Disturbance related to hyperactivity
Alterations in Thought Process related to flight of ideas, delusions, or hallucinations
Impaired Verbal Communication related to pressured speech
Potential Fluid Volume Deficit related to altered sodium excretion secondary to lithium therapy
Noncompliance related to feelings of no longer requiring medication
Knowledge Deficit: (specify)
  examples:
    condition
    pharmacologic therapy

CHILDHOOD BEHAVIORAL DISORDERS (Attention Deficit Disorders, Learning Disabilities)

Alteration in Thought Process related to inattention and impulsivity
Impaired Social Interactions related to inattention, impulsivity, or hyperactivity
Ineffective Individual Coping related to
  examples:
    temper outbursts
    negativism
    mood lability
    stubborness
Grieving (parental): denial, anger, depression related to the anticipated losses secondary to the condition

Alteration in Family Process related to the adjustment requirements for the situation
examples:
- time
- energy
- financial
- physical care
- prognosis

Potential for Violence related to impaired ability to control aggression
Potential Impaired Home Maintenance Management related to inadequate resources, inadequate, housing or impaired caregivers
Potential Social Isolation (child, family) related to the disability and the requirements for the caregivers
Potential Alteration in Parenting: abuse, rejection or overprotection related to inadequate resources or inadequate coping mechanisms
Disturbance in Self-Concept related to the effects of limitations on achievement of developmental tasks

PARANOID DISORDERS

Impaired Social Interactions related to feelings of mistrust and suspicions of others
Ineffective Individual Coping: denial, projection related to inability to accept own feelings and responsibility for actions secondary to low self-esteem
Potential Alteration in Nutrition: Less than Body Requirements related to reluctance to eat secondary to fear of poisoning
Alteration in Thought Processes related to inability to evaluate reality secondary to feelings of mistrust
Social Isolation related to fear and mistrust of situations and others

PERSONALITY DISORDERS

examples:
- schizoid
- antisocial
- borderline
- narcissistic
- avoidant
- compulsive
- histrionic
- passive–aggressive
- paranoid
- schizotypal
- dependent

Ineffective Individual Coping: passive dependence related to subordinating one's needs to decisions of others

Ineffective Individual Coping:
- inappropriate intense anger
- lack of impulse control
- marked mood shifts
- habitual disregard for social norms
- related to altered ability to meet responsibilities (role, social)

Impaired Social Interaction related to inability to maintain enduring attachments secondary to negative responses

Ineffective Individual Coping related to resistance (procrastination, stubbornness, intentional inefficiency) in responses to responsibilities (role, social)

SCHIZOPHRENIC DISORDERS

Alteration in Thought Processes: delusion, hallucinations related to inability to evaluate reality

Potential for Violence to Self or to Others related to responding to delusional thoughts or hallucinations

Impaired Verbal Communications related to incoherent/illogical speech pattern, poverty of content of speech, and side effects of medications

Impaired Social Interactions related to

examples:
- withdrawal from external world
- preoccupation with egocentric and illogical ideas
- inappropriate affect
- inappropriate movements
- extreme suspiciousness

Anxiety related to inability to cope with internal/external stressors

Impaired Home Maintenance Management related to impaired judgement, inability to self-initiate activity, and loss of skills over long course of illness

SOMATOFORM DISORDERS (Somatization, Hypochondriasis, Conversion Reactions)

See also Affective Disorders if indicated.

Impaired Social Interactions related to the effects of multiple somatic complaints on relationships
Ineffective Individual Coping related to unrealistic fear of having a disease despite reassurance to contrary
Anxiety related to somatic complaints and beliefs of having a disease
Ineffective Individual Coping: depression related to belief of not getting proper care or sufficient response from others for complaints
Ineffective Family Coping related to chronicity of illness
Noncompliance related to impaired judgements and thought disturbances
Self-Care Deficit: Dressing/Grooming related to loss of skills, and lack of interest in body and appearance
Social Isolation related to withdrawal from environment
Diversional Activity Deficit related to apathy, inability to initiate goal-directed activities, and loss of skills
Disturbance in Self-Concept related to feelings of worthlessness and lack of ego boundaries
Knowledge Deficit: (specify)
examples:
condition
pharmacologic therapy
tardive dyskinesia
occupational skills
social skills

SUBSTANCE ABUSE DISORDERS

Alteration in Nutrition: Less than Body Requirements related to anorexia
Potential Fluid Volume Deficit related to abnormal fluid loss secondary to vomiting and diarrhea
Potential for Injury related to disorientation, tremors, or impaired judgement
Potential for Violence to self related to disorientation, tremors, or impaired judgement

Potential for Violence related to
examples:
impulsive behavior
disorientation
tremors
impaired judgement

Sleep Pattern Disturbances related to irritability, tremors, and nightmares

Anxiety related to loss of control

Ineffective Individual Coping: anger, dependence, or denial related to inability to constructively manage stressors without drugs/alcohol

Sensory Perceptual Alterations related to:
examples:
confusion
memory losses
impaired judgements
overdose/withdrawal

Disturbance in Self-Concept related to guilt, mistrust, or ambivalence

Impaired Social Interactions related to
examples:
emotional immaturity
irritability
high anxiety
impulsive behavior
aggressive responses

Social Isolation related to loss of work or withdrawal from others

Sexual Dysfunction related to impotence/loss of libido secondary to altered self-concept and substance abuse

Alteration in Family Processes related to disruption in marital dyad and inconsistent limit setting

Knowledge Deficit: (specify)
examples:
condition
treatments available
high-risk situations
community resources

Diagnostic and Therapeutic Procedures

Angioplasty
Percutaneous Transluminal Coronary

Anticoagulant Therapy
Arteriogram
Cardiac Catheterization
Casts
Chemotherapy
Corticosteroid Therapy
Gastrostomy
Hemodialysis
Hemodynamic Monitoring
Hickman Catheter
Intra-aortic Balloon Pumping
Mechanical Ventilation
Pacemaker Insertion
Peritoneal Dialysis
Radiation Therapy (External)
Total Parenteral Nutrition (Hyperalimentation)

ANGIOPLASTY (Percutaneous, Transluminal, Coronary)

Preprocedure Period:

Knowledge Deficit: (specify)
examples:
procedure
preparation
postprocedure care

Anxiety/Fear related to procedure, outcome, and possible need for cardiac surgery

Postprocedure Period:

Potential Complications:
Arrhythmias
Acute coronary occlusion (clot, spasm, collapse)
Myocardial infarction
Arterial dissection or rupture
Hemorrhage/hematoma (site)

Impaired Physical Mobility related to prescribed immobility and restricted movement of involved extremity

Knowledge Deficit: (specify)
examples:
condition
home activities
diet
medications
signs and symptoms of complications

ANTICOAGULANT THERAPY

Potential Complications:
  Hemorrhage
Knowledge Deficit: (specify)
  examples:
    administration schedule
    identification band/card
    contraindications
      food
      medications
    signs and symptoms of bleeding
      skin
      GI
      neurological
    potential hazards
      surgery
      pregnancy
      dental extraction
      shaving

ARTERIOGRAM

Preprocedure Period

Knowledge Deficit: (specify)
  examples:
    procedure
      equipment
      possible sensations
    preparation
    post-care

Postprocedure Period

Potential Complications:
  Hematoma formation
  Parathesia
  Hemorrhage

CARDIAC CATHETERIZATION

Preprocedure Period

Knowledge Deficit: (specify)
  examples:
    procedure
      purpose
      appearance of laboratory positioning
      equipment
      length of
      possible sensations

preparation
NPO
premedication
postprocedure care (frequent versus activity restriction)
Anxiety/Fear related to being awake during the procedure

Postprocedure Period

Potential Complications:
Systemic (hypo/hypervolemia, allergic reaction)
Cardiac (arrhythmias, myocardial infarction, perforation)
Cerebrovascular accident
Neurovascular (hematoma formation [*site*], *hemorrhage* [*site*], *paresis, or parathesia)*
Alteration in Comfort related to tissue trauma and prescribed postprocedure immobilization

CASTS

Potential Complications:
Pressure (edema, mechanical)
Compartmental syndrome
Ulcer formation
Infection
Potential for Injury related to hazards of crutch walking and impaired mobility secondary to cast
Potential Impairment of Skin Integrity related to pressure of cast on skin surface
Potential Impaired Home Maintenance Management related to the restrictions that the cast imposes on performing activities of daily living and role responsibilities
Self-Care Deficits: (specify) related to limitation of movement secondary to cast
Potential Alteration in Respiratory Function related to imposed immobility or restricted respiratory movement secondary to the cast (body)
Diversional Activity Deficit Related to boredom and inability to perform usual recreational activities
Knowledge Deficit: (specify)
examples:
crutch-walking
cast care
exercise program

signs and symptoms of complications
- numbness
- tingling
- burning
- blanching
- cyanosis
- inability to move distal parts
- odor or pain

CHEMOTHERAPY

See also Cancer (General).

Potential Complications:
- *Necrosis/phlebitis at IV site*
- *Thrombocytopenia*
- *Anemia*
- *Leukopenia*
- *Peripheral nerve toxicitus*
- *Anaphylaxis*
- *Pulmonary fibrosis*
- *Central nervous system toxicity*

Potential Fluid Volume Deficit related to gastrointestinal fluid losses secondary to vomiting

Alteration in Nutrition: Less than Body Requirements related to anorexia, nausea, and altered taste sensations

Potential for Infection related to altered immune system secondary to the effects of cytotoxic agents or the disease process

Activity Intolerance related to fatigue

Potential Alteration in Family Processes related to the interruptions that the treatment and schedule have on patterns of living

Potential Sexual Dysfunction related to amenorrhea and sterility (temporary/permanent) secondary to the effects of chemotherapy on testes/ovaries

Potential for Injury related to bleeding tendencies

Alteration in Bowel Elimination: Constipation/Diarrhea related to decreased bowel activity or irritation of epithelium of bowel

Alteration in Oral Mucous Membrane related to irritation of mucosa from medication

CORTICOSTEROID THERAPY

Potential Complications:
- *Peptic ulcer*
- *Diabetes mellitus*
- *Osteoporosis*
- *Hypertension*
- *Thromboembolism*
- *Hypokalemia*

Potential Fluid Volume Excess: edema related to sodium and water retention

Potential for Infection related to immunosuppression secondary to excessive adrenocortical hormones
Potential Alteration in Nutrition: More than Body Requirements related to increased appetite
Disturbance in Self-Concept related to appearance changes (*e.g.*, abnormal fat distribution, increased production of androgens)
Knowledge Deficit: (specify)
examples:
administration schedule
indications for therapy
side effects
signs and symptoms of complications
hazards of adrenal insufficiency
potential causes of adrenal insufficiency
injuries
surgery
vomiting
abrupt cessation of therapy
emergency kit
dietary requirements
prevention of infection

GASTROSTOMY

Potential Complications: gastrointestinal bleeding

Potential for Infection related to gastrostomy incision and enzymatic action of gastric juices on skin
Alteration in Comfort: Pain related to incision and tension on gastrostomy tube
Potential Alteration in Nutrition: Less than Body Requirements related to intake dependent on gastrostomy feedings
Potential Disturbance in Self-Concept related to inability to taste or swallow food/liquids
Knowledge Deficit: (specify)
examples:
nutritional requirements
home care
signs and symptoms of complications
infection
weight loss
nonpatent gastrostomy tube
diarrhea

HEMODIALYSIS

See also Chronic Renal Failure.

Potential Complications (During/Posttreatment):

- *Fluid imbalances (disequilibrium syndrome)*
- *Electrolyte imbalance (potassium, sodium)*
- *Nausea/vomiting*
- *Transfusion reaction*
- *Aneurysm*
- *Hemorrhage*
- *Vascular access (fistula, graft, shunts, venous catheters)*
- *Bleeding*
- *Dialysate leakage*
- *Clots*
- *Disconnection*
- *Infection*
- *Hepatitis B*
- *Fever/chills*

Potential for Injury to (vascular) access site related to vulnerability

Potential for Infection related to direct access to blood stream secondary to vascular access

Powerlessness related to the need for treatments to live despite the effects on life-style

Alteration in Family Processes related to the interruptions of treatment schedule on role responsibilities

Knowledge Deficit: (specify)

- examples:
  - rationale of treatment
  - access site
    - care (general, posttreatment)
    - precautions
    - emergency treatments (disconnected, bleeding, clotting)
  - pretreatment instructions
    - dietary
    - medications
  - assessments
    - bruit
    - weights
    - blood pressure

HEMODYNAMIC MONITORING

See also Medical Diagnosis of the individual.

Potential Complications:

- *Sepsis*
- *Hemorrhage (site)*
- *Emboli*
- *Thrombosis (clotting)*

Bleeding back
Vasospasm
Tissue ischemia/hypoxia
System problems (leaks, air bubbles, misconnection, damaged/unbalanced transducer, damaged amplifier, damaged stopcock, flush device, or pressure tubing)

Potential for Infection related to direct access to blood stream

Impaired Physical Mobility related to the position restrictions during monitoring

Knowledge Deficit: (specify)
examples:
purpose
procedure
associated care

HICKMAN CATHETER

Potential Complications:
Air embolism
Nonpatent catheter

Potential for Infection related to direct access to blood stream

Potential Impaired Home Maintenance Management related to lack of knowledge of catheter management

INTRA AORTIC BALLOON PUMPING

Preprocedure Period

Knowledge Deficit: (specify)
examples:
procedure (preparation)
nursing care

Intra/Post Period

Potential Complications:
Death
Arterial insufficiency/thrombosis
Sepsis/infection
Peripheral neuropathy/claudication
Thrombocytopenia
Bleeding
Emboli
Gastrointestinal bleeding
Disseminated intravascular coagulation
Mechanical malfunction
Arrhythmias

Impaired Physical Mobility related to prescribed immobility and restricted movement of involved extremity
Potential for Infection related to direct access to blood stream
Potential Alteration in Bowel Elimination: Constipation related to immobility and restricted movement of involved limb
Potential Sensory Perceptual Alterations related to:
examples:
immobility
pain
excessive environmental stimuli
disruption of biorhythms
Anxiety/Fear related to treatments, environment, and risk of death
Alteration in Family Processes related to the critical nature of the situation and uncertain prognosis

Mechanical Ventilation

Potential Complications:
Acidosis/alkalosis
Disconnected ventilator
Airway obstruction/atelectasis
Tracheal necrosis
Infection
Gastrointestinal bleeding
Tension pneumothorax
Oxygen toxicity
Respirator dependency
Impaired Verbal Communication related to inability to speak secondary to intubation
Potential Impairment of Skin Integrity related to imposed immobility
Potential for Infection related to the disruption of the skin layer secondary to tracheostomy
Alteration in Family Process related to the critical nature of the situation and uncertain prognosis
Anxiety/Fear related to the condition, treatments, environment, and risk of death
Potential Sensory Perceptual Alterations related to the excessive environmental stimuli and decreased input

of meaningful stimuli secondary to the treatment and the critical care unit

Powerlessness related to respirator dependency

PACEMAKER INSERTION

Preprocedure Period

Knowledge Deficit: (specify)
- examples:
  - procedure
    - purpose
    - appearance of operating room/laboratory
    - positioning
    - equipment
    - possible sensations
  - preparation
    - skin preparation
    - premedication
    - NPO
  - postprocedure
    - X-rays
    - ECG
    - vital signs
    - monitoring
    - activity restrictions
    - site care

Postprocedure Period

Potential Complications:
- *Cardiac (perforation, arrhythmias)*
- *Pacemaker (failure, electromagnetic interference, under/oversensing, partial/improper sensing or wire break)*
- *Rejection of unit*
- *Pressure necrosis of skin over unit*
- *Site (hemorrhage, infection)*

Alteration in Comfort related to pain at insertion site and prescribed postprocedure immobilization

Potential Alteration in Respiratory Function related to imposed immobility postprocedure

Potential for Infection related to operative site

Knowledge Deficit: (specify)
- examples:
  - site care
  - signs and symptoms of skin complications

electromagnetic interference
- microwave ovens
- arc welding equipment
- gasoline engines
- electric motors
- antitheft devices
- power transmitters

pacemaker function
- daily pulse taking
- signs of impending battery failure

activity restrictions
follow-up care

PERITONEAL DIALYSIS

Potential Complications:
- *Fluid imbalances*
- *Electrolyte imbalances*
- *Hemorrhage*
- *Negative nitrogen balance*
- *Catheter problems (displacement, plugging, fibrin clots)*
- *Bowel/bladder perforation*
- *Hyperglycemia*
- *Peritonitis*

Potential for Infection related to direct access to peritoneal cavity, the need to disconnect catheter for treatment, and growth medium potential of the dialysate (high glucose concentration)

Potential for Injury to catheter site related to vulnerability

Potential Impaired Breathing Patterns related to immobility and pressure on diaphragm during dwell time

Alteration in Comfort related to
examples:
- rapid instillation
- pressure from fluid
- excessive suction during outflow
- extreme temperature of solution (hot or cold)

Potential Alteration in Nutrition: Less than Body Requirements related to anorexia secondary to abdominal distention during dwelling, protein loss in dialysate, or vomiting related to fluid instillation that is too rapid

Potential Fluid Volume Excess related to fluid retention secondary to catheter problems (kinks, blockages) and/or position

Alteration in Family Processes related to the interruptions of treatment schedule on role responsibilities
Powerlessness related to the need for treatment to live despite the effects on life style
Impaired Home Maintenance Management related to lack of knowledge of treatment procedure
Knowledge Deficit: (specify)
- examples:
  - rationale of treatment
  - home care
  - self-care activities
    - protection of catheter
    - aseptic technique
  - activity needs
  - prescribed diet
  - control of fluid intake/output
  - medication regimen
  - signs/symptoms of complications
  - follow-up visits
  - daily recording
    - intake
    - output
    - blood pressure
    - weights

RADIATION THERAPY (External)

Pretherapy Period
- Knowledge Deficit: (specify)
  - examples:
    - procedure
    - site-related, local/systemic effects of therapy (skin gastrointestinal, neurologic, oral membranes)

Posttherapy Period

Potential Complications of Head/Brain Irradiation: Increased intracranial pressure
Potential Impairment of Skin Integrity related to radiation exposure
Disturbance in Self-Concept related to alopecia secondary to irradiation to head and visible markings outlining treatment field

Alteration in Oral Mucous Membrane related to mucosites, gingivites, esophagitis, and dry mouth secondary to irradiation (head/neck, chest/back)
Alteration in Comfort related to nausea and vomiting secondary to irradiation of abdomen/lower back
Alteration in Bowel Elimination: Diarrhea related to increased peristalsis secondary to irradiation of abdomen/lower back
Potential for Infection: skin related to moist skin reaction
Potential Alteration in Nutrition: Less than Body Requirements related to anorexia, nausea/vomiting, or stomatitis
Activity Intolerance related to fatigue secondary to treatments or transportation
Knowledge Deficit: (specify)
examples:
skin care
signs of complications

TOTAL PARENTERAL NUTRITION
(Hyperalimentation Therapy)

Potential Complications:
Infection
Hypo- /hyperglycemia
Air embolism
Perforation
Pneumo-, hydro-, hemothorax

Potential for Infection related to catheter's direct access to blood stream
Potential Impairment of Skin Integrity related to continuous skin surface irritation secondary to catheter and adhesive
Potential Disturbance in Self-Concept related to inability to ingest food
Potential Alteration in Oral Mucous Membrane related to inability to ingest food/fluids
Knowledge Deficit: (specify)
examples:
home care
signs and symptoms of complications
catheter care
follow-up care (laboratory studies)

Appendix: Data-Base Assessment Guide

This guide directs the nurse to collect data to assess functional health patterns* of the individual and to determine the presence of actual, potential, or possible nursing diagnoses. Should the person have medical problems, the nurse will also have to assess additional data in order to collaborate with the physician in monitoring the problem.

As with any printed assessment tool, the nurse must determine whether to collect or defer certain data. The symbol Δ identifies data that should be collected on hospitalized persons. The collection of data in sections not marked with Δ probably should be deferred with most acutely ill persons or when the information is irrelevant to the particular individual.

Data-Base Assessment Format

1. Health perception–health management pattern

   "How would you usually describe your health?"

Excellent	Fair
Good	Poor

   "How would you describe your health at this time?"

   "What do you do to keep healthy and to prevent disorders in yourself? In your children?"

* The functional health patterns have been adapted from Gordon M: Nursing Diagnosis: Application and Process. New York, McGraw-Hill, 1982

- Adequate nutrition
- Weight control
- Exercise program
- Self-exams (breast, testicular)
- Professional exams (gynecological, dental)
- Immunizations

△ Reason for and expectations of hospitalization (and previous hospital experiences)

△ "Describe your illness"

- Cause
- Onset

△ "What treatments or practices have been prescribed?"

- Diet
- Weight loss
- Medications
- Surgery
- Cessation of smoking
- Exercises

△ "Have you been able to follow the prescribed instructions?" If not, "What has prevented you?"

△ "Have you experienced or do you anticipate a problem with caring for yourself (your children, your home)?"

- Mobility problems
- Sensory deficits (vision, hearing)
- Financial concerns
- Structural barriers (stairs, narrow doorways)

2. △ Nutritional-metabolic pattern

"What is the usual daily food intake (meals, snacks)?"

"What is the usual fluid intake (type, amounts)?"

"How is your appetite?"

- Indigestion
- Nausea
- Vomiting
- Sore mouth

"What are your food restrictions or preferences?"

"Any supplements (vitamins, feedings)?"

"Has your weight changed in the last 6 months?" If yes, "Why?"

"Any problems with ability to eat?"

- Swallow liquids
- Swallow solids
- Chew
- Feed self

3. △ Elimination pattern

Bladder

"Are there any problems or complaints with the usual pattern of urinating?"

- Oliguria
- Polyuria
- Dysuria
- Dribbling
- Retention
- Burning
- Incontinence

"Are assistive devices used?"

- Intermittent catheterization
- Catheter (Foley, external)
- Incontinent briefs
- Cystostomy

Bowel

"What is the usual time, frequency, color, consistency, pattern?"

"Assistive devices (type, frequency)?"

- Ileostomy
- Colostomy
- Enemas
- Cathartics
- Laxatives
- Suppositories

Skin

"What is the skin condition?"

- Color, temperature, turgor
- Lesions (type, description, location)
- Edema (type, location)
- Pruritus (location)

4. Activity-exercise pattern

"Describe usual daily/weekly activities of daily living"

- Occupation
- Leisure activities
- Exercise pattern (type, frequency)

△ "Are there any limitations in ability?"

- Ambulating (gait, weight-bearing, balance)
- Bathing self (shower, tub)
- Dressing/grooming (oral hygiene)
- Toileting (commode, toilet, bedpan)

"Are there complaints of dyspnea or fatigue?"

5. △ Sleep-rest pattern
   "What is the usual sleep pattern?"
   - Bedtime
   - Hours slept
   - Sleep aids (medication, food)
   - Sleep routine

   "Any problems?"
   - Difficulty falling asleep
   - Difficulty remaining asleep
   - Not feeling rested after sleep
6. △ Cognitive-perceptual pattern
   "Any deficits in sensory perception (hearing, sight, touch)?"
   - Glasses
   - Hearing aid

   "Any complaints?"
   - Vertigo
   - Insensitivity to superficial pain
   - Insensitivity to cold or heat

   "Able to read and write?"
7. Self-perception pattern
   - △ "What are you most concerned about?"
   - "What are your present health goals?"
   - △ "How would you describe yourself?"
   - "Has being ill made you feel differently about yourself?"
   - "To what do you attribute the following?"
     - Becoming ill
     - Getting better
     - Maintaining health
8. Role-relationship pattern
   - △ Communication
   - What language is spoken?
   - Is speech clear? Relevant?
   - Assess ability to express self and understand others (verbally, in writing, with gestures)
   - Relationships
   - "Do you live alone?" "If not, with whom?"
   - "Who do you turn to for help in time of need?"
   - Assess family life (members, educational level, occupations)
     - Cultural background
     - Activities (lone or group)
     - Roles discipline
     - Decision-making
     - Communication patterns
     - Finances

"Any complaints?"

Parenting difficulties
Difficulties with relative (in-laws, parents)
Marital difficulties
Abuse (physical, verbal, substance)

9. Sexuality-sexual functioning

"Has there been or do you anticipate a change in your sexual relations because of your condition?"

Fertility
Libido
Erections
Menstruation
Pregnancy
Contraceptives
History

Assess knowledge of sexual functioning

10. Coping–stress management pattern

△ "How do you make decisions (alone, with assistance, who)?"

△ "Has there been a loss in your life in the past year (or changes—moves, job, health)?"

"What do you like about yourself?"

"What would you like to change in your life?"

"What is preventing you?"

"What do you do when you are tense or under stress (*e.g.*, problem-solve, eat, sleep, take medication, seek help)?"

△ "What can the nurses do to provide you with more comfort and security during your hospitalization?"

11. Value-belief system

"With what (whom) do you find a source of strength or meaning?"

"Is religion or God important to you?"

"What are your religious practices (type, frequency)?"

"Have your values or moral beliefs been challenged recently? Describe."

△ "Is there a religious person or practice (diet, book, ritual) that you would desire during hospitalization (institutionalization)?"

12. △ Physical assessment (objective)

General appearance
Weight and height
Eyes (appearance, drainage)

- Pupils (size, equal, reactive to light)
- Vision (glasses)

Mouth

- Mucous membrane (color, moisture, lesions)
- Teeth (condition, loose, broken, dentures)

Hearing (hearing aids)

Pulses (radial, apical, peripheral)

- Rate, rhythm, volume

Respirations

- Rate, quality, breath sounds (upper and lower lobes)

Blood pressure

Bowel sounds

Temperature

Skin (color, temperature, turgor)

- Lesions, edema, pruritus

Functional ability (mobility and safety)

- Dominant hand
- Use of right and left hands, arms, legs
- Strength, grasp
- Range of motion
- Gait (stability)
- Use of aids (wheelchair, braces, cane, walker)
- Weight-bearing (full, partial, none)

Mental status

- Orientation (time, place, person, events)
- Memory
- Affect
- Eye contact

Index

abdominal aortic aneurysm resection, 136–137
abdominoperineal resection, 135–136
ABO incompatibility, 170
abortion
  induced, 158–159
  spontaneous, 159
abruptio placentae, 160
acquired immune deficiency syndrome (AIDS), 129
Activity Intolerance, 3–4
acute respiratory distress syndrome (ARDS), 91
Addison's disease, 94
adjustment disorders, 197–198
adolescent/pediatric disorders, 172–194
advice, health-related, deviation from, 44–45
affective disorders, 195–196
age-related conditions, primary and secondary prevention for, 30–36
aggressive behavior, 79–80
AIDS. *See* acquired immune deficiency syndrome
Airway Clearance, Ineffective, 56–57
aldosteronism, primary, 95
aloneness
  creative, 70
  negative state of, 70
Alzheimer's disease, 112
amputation, 136
amyotrophic lateral sclerosis, 110–112
anal fissure, 102, 137–138
anemia, 86–87
  aplastic, 87
  pernicious, 87
  sickle cell, 193
aneurysm resection, 136–137
angina pectoris, 84
angioplasty, 203
ankle replacement, 138–139
anorectal surgery, 137–138
anorexia nervosa, 196–197
anticoagulant therapy, 204
Anxiety, 5–6
anxiety states, 197–198
aplastic anemia, 87
ARDS. *See* acute respiratory distress syndrome
arterial occlusion, with graft of lower extremity, 138
arteriography, 204
arthritis, rheumatoid, juvenile, 191
arthroplasty, 138–139
arthroscopy, 139–140
arthrotomy, 139–140
assessment guide, data-base, 215–220
asthma, 174
attention deficit disorders, 198–199

back, low, pain in, 125
battered child syndrome, 176–177
behavioral disorders, childhood, 198–199
belief system, disturbance in, 72–73
bipolar disorder, 198
bladder tumor, transurethral resection in, 154
bleeding, uterine, during pregnancy, 160
blood supply, capillary
  decrease in, 75–77
  decreased tissue perfusion in, 75–77
body image, change in, 60–62
boredom, statements of, 19
Bowel Elimination, Alteration in, 7–10
brain tumor, 107–108
Breathing Patterns, Ineffective, 57
bronchitis, 91–92
bunionectomy, 139–140
burns, 120–122

calculi, renal, 107
cancer, 130–132
  colon/rectal, 132
cardiac catheterization, 204–205
cardiac conditions, 84–86
cardiac disease, prenatal and postpartum, 163
Cardiac Output: Decreased, Alteration in, 10–12
cardiovascular/hematologic/peripheral vascular disorders, 83–91

carotid endarterectomy, 140
casts, 205–206
cataracts, 116–117
catheter, Hickman, 209
catheterization, cardiac, 204–205
celiac disease, 174–175
cellulitis, pelvic, 165
cerebral palsy, 175–176
cerebral vascular accident, 108–110
cesarean section, 140
chemotherapy, 206
child abuse, 176–177
child neglect, 176–177
childhood behavioral disorders, 198–199
cholecystectomy, 140–141
chronic illness, developmental problems/needs related to, 173–174
chronic obstructive pulmonary disease (COPD), 91–92
cirrhosis, 95–96
cleft lip, 178
cleft palate, 178
CMV. *See* cytomegalovirus
coagulation, disseminated intravascular (DIC), 88
cognitive knowledge, deficiency in, 42–43
colon, cancer of, 132
colostomy, 135–136
Comfort, Alteration in: Pain, 12–13
communicable diseases, 178–179
Communication, Impaired Verbal, 13–15
congestive heart failure, with pulmonary edema, 84–85
connective tissue disorders, 122–127
constipation, 7–8
control, personal, perception of lack of, 51–52
conversion reactions, 201
convulsive disorders, 179
COPD. *See* chronic obstructive pulmonary disease
Coping
  Ineffective Family, 17–19
  Ineffective Individual, 15–17
coronary artery bypass, 144–145
corticosteroid therapy, 206–207
cranial surgery, 141
Cushing's syndrome, 96
cystic fibrosis, 179–180
cystitis, 106
cystostomy, suprapubic, 154–155
cytomegalovirus (CMV), congenital, 168

D&C. *See* dilatation and curettage
data-base assessment guide, 215–220
deep vein thrombosis, 89
degenerative disorders, 110–112
dehydration, 23–25
dementia, presenile, 112
demyelinating disorders, 110–112
depression, 195–196
dermatitis, 119
dermatologic disorders, 119
detached retina, 116–117
developmental problems/needs, related to chronic illness, 173–174
diabetes mellitus
  adult, 97–98
  neonate of mother with, 168–169
  postpartum, 164
  prenatal, 163–164
diagnostic and therapeutic procedures, 202–214
diagnostic categories
  medical, 83–214
  nursing, 3–80
diarrhea, 8–10
DIC. *See* disseminated intravascular coagulation
dilatation and curettage (D&C), 141
disseminated intravascular coagulation (DIC), 88
Diversional Activity Deficit, 19
diverticulitis, 103
diverticulosis, 103
Down's syndrome, 180–181
Duchenne's muscular dystrophy, 186–187

ectopic pregnancy, 159
eczema, 119
elimination, bowel, alterations in, 7–10
embolism, pulmonary, 93
emphysema, 91–92
encephalitis, 128–129
endocarditis, 85

endometriosis, 164–165
endometritis, 165
enteritis, regional, 103
epilepsy, 112–113
esophageal disorders, 102
esophagitis, 102

failure to thrive, 181
Family Processes, Alteration in, 20–21
family(ies)
ineffective coping by, 17–19
maintenance of, in safe home environment, difficulty in, 37–38
at risk for parenting difficulties, 50
Fear, 21–23
fetal death, 163
fluid overload, 25–26
Fluid Volume
Deficit, 23–25
Excess, 25–26
food intake
excess, weight gain in, 47–48
inadequate, reduced weight in, 46–47
fractures, 123–124
fungal infections, of skin, 120

Gas Exchange, Impaired, 57–58
gastroenteritis, 102
gastrointestinal disorders, 101–104
gastrostomy, 207
glaucoma, 116–117
glomerular disorders, 182
glomerulonephritis, 106, 182
graft, arterial, arterial occlusion and, 138
Graves' disease, 99
Grieving, 27–28
Guillain-Barré syndrome, 110–112
gynecologic conditions, 164–165

Health Maintenance, Alteration in, 28–37
heart failure, congestive, with pulmonary edema, 84–85
hematologic conditions, 86–89
hemodialysis, 208
hemodynamic monitoring, 208–209
hemophilia, 183
hemorrhoids, 102, 137–138
hepatitis, 98
herpes, 129
congenital, 168
herpes zoster, 120
hiatal hernia, 102
Hickman catheter, 209
hip
fractured, 141–142
replacement, total, 138–139
Home Maintenance Management, Impaired, 37–38
Huntington's disease, 112
hydatidiform mole, 160
hyperalimentation therapy, 214
hyperbilirubinemia, 170
hyperemesis gravidarum, 159
hypertension, 89
hyperthyroidism, 99
hypochondriasis, 201
hypothermia, severe, 120–122
hypothyroidism, 99
hysterectomy, 142

ileal conduit, 154–155
ileostomy, 135–136
illness, chronic, developmental problems/needs related to, 173–174
immune deficiency syndrome, acquired (AIDS), 129
immunodeficient disorders, 127–129
impetigo, 120
infant(s). *See* neonate(s)
Infection(s)
congenital, 168
optic, 117–118
Potential for, 38–40
reproductive tract, 165
respiratory tract, lower, 190
skin, 120
urinary tract, 106
infectious disorders, 127–129
infectious mononucleosis, 183–184
inflammation(s)
intestinal, 103
of nervous system, 110–112
ophthalmic, 116–117
Injury, Potential for, 40–41
integumentary disorders, 118–122

intestinal disorders, inflammatory, 103
intra-aortic balloon pumping, 209–210

jaw, fractured, 123

knee replacement, 138–139
Knowledge Deficit, 42–43

Laennec's cirrhosis, 95–96
laminectomy, 143
laryngectomy, 149–150
learning disabilities, 198–199
Legg-Calvé-Perthes disease, 184
leukemia, 184–185
lip, cleft, 178
loss, responses to, 27–28
low back pain, 125
lupus erythematosus, 127–128

mania, 198
mastectomy, 143–144
mastitis, lactational, 162–163
mastoidectomy, tympanic, 147
mastoiditis, 117–118
mechanical ventilation, 210–211
meningitis, 128–129, 185
meningomyelocele, 185–186
meniscectomy, 139–140
mental activities, disruption in, 73–74
mental retardation, 186
metabolic/endocrine disorders, 93–101
Mobility, Physical, Impaired, 43–44
mononucleosis, infectious, 183–184
multiple sclerosis, 110–112
muscular dystrophy, 110–112, 186–187
musculoskeletal disorders, 122–127
myasthenia gravis, 110–112
myocardial infarction, 86
myocardial revascularization, 144–145
myringotomy, 147
myxedema, 99–100

narcotic-addicted mother, 170–171
neonatal conditions, 165–172
neonate(s)
  death of, 163
  of diabetic mother, 168–169
  high-risk, 169
    family of, 169–170
  large for gestation age (LGA), 167–168
  of narcotic-addicted mother, 170–171
  normal, 166
  postmature, 167–168
  premature, 167
  small for gestation age (SGA), 167–168
  with special problem, 168
neoplastic disorders, 129–132
nephrectomy, 150
nephrostomy, percutaneous, 150
nephrotic syndrome, 182
nervous system disorders, 110–112
neurologic disorders, 107–116
noncompliance (specify), 44–45
nutrition
  Alteration in
    Less than requirements, 46–47
    More than requirements, 47–48
  total parenteral, 214

obesity, 100, 187–188
obstetric conditions
  intrapartum period, 161
  postpartum period, 161–163
  prenatal period, 156–158
ophthalmic disorders, 116–117
ophthalmic surgery, 145–147
optic disorders, 117–118
optic surgery, 147
Oral Mucous Membrane, Alteration in, 48–49
osteomyelitis, 125, 188
osteoporosis, 126

pacemaker insertion, 211–212
pain, 12–13
  low back, 125
palate, cleft, 178
pancreatitis, 100–101
paranoid disorders, 199
parasitic disorders, 188–189
Parenting, Alteration in, 49–51
Parkinson's disease, 110–112

pathogenic agent, risk of invasion by, 38–40
pediatric/adolescent disorders, 172–194
pelvic cellulitis, 165
pelvic exenteration, 148
peptic ulcer, 103–104
pericarditis, 85
peripheral vascular conditions, 89–91
peripheral vascular disease, 90
peritoneal dialysis, 212–213
peritonitis, 165
pernicious anemia, 87
personal identity, change in, 60–62
personality disorders, 199–200
phobias, 197–198
physical movement, limitation of, 43–44
placenta previa, 160
pleural effusion, 92
pneumonia, 92–93
poisoning, 189–190
polycythemia vera, 88–89
Powerlessness, 51–52
pregnancy
  concomitant medical conditions in, 163–164
  extrauterine, 159
  uterine bleeding during, 160
premature neonate, 167
presenile dementia, 112
pressure ulcers, 119–120
prevention, primary and secondary, for age-related conditions, 30–36
prostate, disorders of, transurethral resection in, 154
psoriasis, 119
psychiatric disorders, 194–202
psychomotor skills, deficiency in, 42–43
pulmonary disease, chronic obstructive (COPD), 91–92
pulmonary edema, congestive heart failure with, 84–85
pulmonary embolism, 93
pyelonephritis, 106

radial neck dissection, 149–150
radiation therapy, external, 213–214
Rape Trauma Syndrome, 53–54
rectum, cancer of, 132
regional enteritis, 103
renal calculi, 107
renal failure
  acute, 104–105
  chronic, 105–106
renal surgery, 150
renal transplant, 151–152
renal/urinary tract disorders, 104–107
reproductive tract infections, 165
respiratory disorders, 91–93
respiratory distress syndrome, 171
  acute (ARDS), 91
Respiratory Function, Alteration in, 54–58
respiratory tract, lower, infection of, 190
retina, detached, 116–117
Reye's syndrome, 191–192
Rh incompatibility, 170
rheumatic diseases, 126–127
rheumatic fever, 190–191
rheumatoid arthritis, juvenile, 191
role performance, change in, 60–62
rubella, congenital, 168

schizophrenic disorders, 200
sclerosis, amyotrophic lateral, 110–112
scoliosis, 192
seizure disorders, 112–113
self, maintenance of, in safe home environment, difficulty in, 37–38
Self-care Deficit, 58–60
Self-concept, Disturbance in, 60–62
self-esteem, change in, 60–62
sensory disorders, 116–118
Sensory-Perceptual Alteration, 62–63
sepsis, neonatal, 171–172
septicemia, neonatal, 171–172
Sexual Dysfunction, 64–66
sexually transmitted infectious diseases, 129
sickle cell anemia, 193
skin infections, 120
Skin Integrity, Impairment of, 66–67
Sleep Pattern Disturbance, 67–69
Social Interactions, Impaired, 69–70
Social Isolation, 70–72

somatization, 201
somatoform disorders, 201
speech, appropriate, decreased
ability in, 13–15
spinal cord injury, 113–115
Spiritual Distress, 72–73
stapedectomy, 147
stasis ulcers, 90
stimuli, incoming, change in
amount, pattern, or
interpretation of, 62–63
stress disorders, traumatic, 197–198
stressors, inability to manage
by family, 17–19
by individual, 15–17
substance abuse disorders, 201–202
surgery, general
postoperative period in, 134–135
preoperative period in, 134
surgical procedures, 132–155
syphilis, congenital, 168

therapeutic and diagnostic
procedures, 202–214
thermal injuries, 120–122
thoracic surgery, 152
Thought Processes, Alteration in, 73–74
thrive, failure to, 181
thrombangiitis obliterans, 90
thrombosis, deep vein, 89
thyrotoxicosis, 99
Tissue Perfusion, Alteration in, 75–77
tonsillectomy, 153
tonsillitis, 193
total parenteral nutrition, 214
toxemia, 159–160
toxoplasmosis, congenital, 168
transplantation, renal, 151–152
transurethral resection, 154
trauma, optic, 117–118
traumatic stress disorders, 197–198
tumor(s)
bladder, transurethral resection
in, 154
brain, 107–108
tympanic mastoidectomy, 147
tympanoplasty, 147

ulcer(s)
peptic, 103–104
pressure, 119–120
stasis, 90
ulcerative colitis, 103
unconsciousness, 115–116
uremia, 105–106
ureterosigmoidostomy, 154–155
ureterostomy, 154–155
urinary diversion, 154–155
urinary dysfunction, risk of, 77–79
Urinary Elimination, Alteration in Patterns of, 77–79
urinary tract infections, 106
urolithiasis, 107
uterine bleeding during pregnancy,
160
uterus
nonmalignant lesions of, during
pregnancy, 160
rupture of, during pregnancy,
160

vaginitis, 165
value system, disturbance in, 72–73
varicose veins, 90–91
venereal diseases, 129
ventilation, mechanical, 210–211
verbal communication, impaired,
13–15
Violence, Potential for, 79–80

weight
gain, in excess food intake, 47–48
reduced, in inadequate food
intake, 46–47
wellness, state of, disruption in, 28–37
Wilms' tumor, 193–194
words, understanding of, decreased
ability in, 13–15